Margaret E. Mohler, ACSW

2643 Bridgeport Way

Sacramento, Cal.

Nov. 1966

An Approach to
Community
Mental Health

GERALD CAPLAN

M.D., D.P.M.

*Associate Professor of Mental Health and
Director of Community Mental Health Program
Harvard School of Public Health, Boston, Mass.
Formerly, Psychiatrist, Tavistock Clinic, London*

GRUNE & STRATTON

AN APPROACH TO
COMMUNITY MENTAL HEALTH

GRUNE & STRATTON, Inc.
381 Park Avenue South
New York, N.Y. 10016

Printed in U.S.A. (G-A)

CONTENTS

Acknowledgements

Thanks are due to the following for permission to quote material that has already appeared in print: John Bowlby and the Director of Publications, World Health Organization, in respect of *Maternal Care and Mental Health* by John Bowlby; International Universities Press in respect of 'Emotional Inoculation: Theory and Research on Effects of Preparatory Communications' by Irving L. Janis, from *Psychoanalysis and the Social Sciences*; The Milbank Memorial Fund in respect of 'Ingredients of a Rehabilitation Program' by Robert C. Hunt, and 'Hospital Community Relationships' by Duncan Macmillan, from *An Approach to the Prevention of Disability from Chronic Psychoses.*

Introduction

I have entitled this book AN APPROACH TO COMMUNITY MENTAL HEALTH. I use the term 'community mental health' to refer to the processes involved in raising the level of mental health among the people in a community, and in reducing the numbers of those suffering from mental disorders. The term 'mental health' is very difficult to define, and in this introduction I wish merely to indicate that I use it to refer to the potential of a person to solve his problems in a reality-based way within the framework of his traditions and culture. Many people believe that there is a relationship between the capacity for reality-based problem-solving and the likelihood of a person falling ill with a mental disorder, but up to the present there has been no proof of this relationship. Whether it exists or not, I believe that the capacity of a person to deal with his problems in a reality-based way has merit in its own right; and to increase this capacity among the members of a community is a legitimate goal of a community mental health programme.

The second aspect of community mental health activities, namely the reduction in the number of cases of mental disorder in a community, involves us in problems of prevention. In the field of psychiatry and in other fields of medicine, the topic of prevention can be considered under three main headings. First, there is *Primary Prevention*. By this I mean the processes involved in reducing the risk that people in the community will fall ill with mental disorders. The next category of prevention is known as *Secondary Prevention*. I use this term to refer to the activities involved in reducing the duration of established cases of mental disorder and thus reducing their prevalence in the community. Involved here is the prevention of disability by case-finding and early diagnosis and by effective treatment. The last category is known as *Tertiary Prevention*. This means the prevention of defect and crippling among the members of a community. Involved here are rehabilitation services which aim at returning sick people as soon as possible to a maximum degree of effectiveness. I refer from time to time both to Secondary Prevention and to Tertiary Prevention, but the strongest emphasis is placed on the area of Primary Prevention, since this has been until recently a relatively unexplored area in the field of mental health and psychiatry.

The first five chapters of the book are based on lectures delivered at an Institute for Maternal and Child Nursing held at Denver, Colorado, in 1959, under the title 'Community Mental Health Aspects of Maternal and Child Nursing'. These lectures were delivered to an audience drawn from the ranks of nursing education, public health nursing in the field of maternal and child health, and from hospital nursing in the fields of obstetrics and paediatrics. Some of the fruitful discussion that followed these talks has been presented at the end of the relevant chapters.

In the first chapter I have outlined some of the concepts used throughout the book in discussing the primary prevention of mental disorders and I have indicated what I consider to be some fundamental principles involved in planning community programmes of preventive psychiatry.

In the second chapter I have turned my attention to problems of individual personality development and related them to preventive intervention. In particular I have focused on some of the latest thinking in the field of psycho-analytic psychology which has implications for preventive psychiatry.

Chapter 3 is concerned with the psychology of pregnancy, and the origins of mother-child relationships, considered both from a theoretical point of view and also in relation to some of the practical implications for work with pregnant women and their families in prenatal clinics and lying-in hospitals.

Two topics are discussed in Chapter 4. First, under 'Early Mother-Child Relationsihps', I have linked what is known about the development of the bond between mother and child to practical issues of the health supervision of mothers and children in clinics for well babies. Secondly, under 'The Effects of Mother-Child Separation', I have discussed a theme of fundamental importance in the field of maternal and child health which has direct relevance for much of our work in the field.

In Chapter 5 I have described some of the research that we have been carrying out at the Harvard School of Public Health, and some of our early tentative findings that are likely to be significant for community mental health practice.

The remaining chapters derive from addresses I have given to various groups of professional workers. Chapter 6 is based on a paper entitled 'The Mental Hygiene Role of the Nurse in Maternal and Child Care' which was first published in *Nursing Outlook*, Vol. 2, January 1954. Chapter 7 first appeared under the title 'The Role of the Social Worker in Preventive Psychiatry', and is reprinted with the permission of the National Association of Social Workers from *Medical Social Work*, Vol. IV, No. 4, September 1955. Chapter 8 was originally published as 'Practical Steps for the Family Physician in the Prevention of Emotional Disorder' in the *Journal of the American Medical Association*, Vol. 170, p. 1,497, 1959. Chapter 9 is an edited version of a paper that I delivered at the Institute of Community Mental Health, organized by the State Health Department, Honolulu, Hawaii, in 1960. Here I have presented my views on psychiatric programmes as a whole and have indicated how the preventive services described elsewhere in the book fit into the total picture. I have also described how some of the fundamental principles of community mental health and crisis theory can be applied in planning programmes for the treatment and control of established cases of mental disorders.

CHAPTER 1

A Community Approach to Preventive Psychiatry – a Conceptual Framework

DURING the last few years a number of psychiatrists in different parts of the world have been exploring a new approach to the problem of preventing psychiatric illness. Instead of basing themselves solely, as in the past, on the concept of early case-finding, diagnosis, and treatment with the goal of 'nipping in the bud' by radical and rapid methods of therapy cases of incipient disease, these workers have set themselves the additional goal of dealing on a community-wide basis with factors that are thought to be pathogenic, in the hope that this will lead to a reduction in the incidence of psychiatric illness in the population. This approach is complicated by the fact that we have as yet no sure knowledge of the factors that lead to psychiatric pathology. We do not really know what causes mental disorder. At least we only know that in any individual case, not one, but many, complicated inter-related factors are responsible for the psychopathological resolution – factors based on constitution, early childhood experiences, vicissitudes of instinctual development, and later socio-cultural pressures.

Our lack of knowledge in regard to the significance of the different factors has to be remedied by a continuation of existing research into aetiology. But, meanwhile, preventive psychiatrists have been able to learn a lesson from their public health colleagues in regard to the handling of the problem of the multifactorial nature of the picture.

The incidence of cases of clinical tuberculosis, for example, in any community is no longer conceived of in public health circles as being merely dependent upon the single factor of the presence or absence of the tubercle bacillus. It is recognized that there are many complicated issues that will determine whether a particular person exposed to the germ will contract the clinical disease: issues involving virulence of the germ, host susceptibility, and various environmental factors. Many of these factors are either unknown or not easily ascertainable in a community, but this does not prevent the public health man from being able to plan and carry out very effective control programmes to reduce clinical tuberculosis in his area; and a good proportion of his programme is not focused at all on the attempt to eradicate the tubercle bacillus itself. The fundamental principle upon which he operates is to conceive of the human community as living in an ecological equilibrium with the community of tubercle bacilli; and then to attempt to move this equilibrium in a healthy direction, as far as the people are concerned, by dealing with those forces which are accessible to his manipulation. The important point is that by altering a significant proportion of the forces he swings the whole equilibrium over to the healthy side. A similar approach governs some of the recent attempts in community-oriented preventive psychiatry. Whether it will have as happy an outcome in the field of mental health as has been achieved by our public health colleagues in the field of physical health remains to be seen. At the moment we are still in the stages of the earliest fumbling attempts. I shall describe some of these so that the reader may judge whether we are moving in the right direction, or whether other approaches might prove fruitful.

In pursuit of the goal of altering what we think are unhealthy forces in a community from the point of view of the mental health, either present or future, of the population, we have been operating in two main ways, which I have called, on the one hand, *Administrative Action,* and, on the other hand, *Personal Interaction.* I shall describe a few examples of each of these to indicate what I have in mind.

ADMINISTRATIVE ACTION

The goal here is to reduce preventable stress, or to provide services to assist people facing stress to healthier problem-solving, by means of governmental or other administrative action. The object is to influence laws, statutes, regulations, and customs, in order to achieve these ends. It is recognized that what is involved is specific culture change; and since all cultures are to be conceived of as systems of interdependent forces, we realize we must move cautiously lest a favourable change in one area of the system may lead to unexpected unfavourable side-effects in other parts. The system is interdependent – alteration of any one part affects the whole. It may be thought desirable to alter some particular aspect in order to achieve some mental health goal, but something else may happen that was entirely unforeseen and may leave things worse off in the end than they were in the beginning.

Despite this danger, which has not always been clearly borne in mind by those of us who have engaged in this type of work, we have, during the past few years, built up a body of experience which indicates that this may be a promising avenue for exploration.

The role of the mental health specialist in this type of work is to act as the consultant and adviser to administrative and governmental bodies. He seeks to introduce a point of view to the administrators that is dependent upon his own specialized knowledge of interpersonal forces and, in particular, upon his knowledge of the psychological needs of individuals and groups. His goal is that the emerging plan or regulation will take account of the mental health needs of the total community, and that at least it will not add to the mental health burdens.

In England

One example of this work, from England, is John Bowlby's studies on the pathogenic influence of prolonged mother-child separation in early childhood on the child's personality development. Although Bowlby has not yet proved his case, and, indeed, some of his latest research results are far from conclusive, many

3

of us with clinical experience in this field agree that, other things being equal, prolonged separation of mother and child is not a good thing. The interesting point is that even before Bowlby has proved his case and certainly before he has teased out more than a small proportion of the interrelated forces involved, he has been able to influence the policy of the Ministry of Health so that one source of mother-child separation has been radically reduced over the whole country. In 1952 a directive was issued by the Ministry to all hospitals with children's wards to the effect that wherever possible daily visiting of children by their parents was to be permitted and encouraged. Recent figures show that by 1960 about 80 to 90 per cent of the children's wards and institutions were carrying out this directive. A revolutionary and powerful blow for the cause of mental health in childhood was struck by that regulation. It is too early to see what the side-effects have been in regard to compensatory forces set up among the nurses and the administrators of children's institutions. These will certainly have to be carefully watched. What is involved here is a major change in the culture of the child-caring institutions. But already in the past eight years, the incidence of mother-child separation in England has been drastically reduced.

In Israel

Another example comes from Israel. When I first went there in 1948 there began a tremendous wave of immigration into the country. In the twelve years since the establishment of the State in 1948, the population of the country has more than doubled. For a number of reasons the immigrants were originally housed on arrival in huge camps in large army-style barrack huts. Each hut housed 30 to 50 people. There was no provision for privacy, no segregation of family units, and minimal facilities for work. Food was provided in communal dining-halls. The immigrants stayed in these camps for many months until arrangements could be made to transfer them to permanent settlements. By that time many of them had sunk into an apathetic dependent state, and when the opportunity for independent and self-respecting work arrived many could not grasp it.

4

I remember very vividly the complaints and the grumbles of the government administrators responsible for this immigrant programme when they said, 'We do all that we can for these people, and then when we give them a chance to settle on the land and do some useful work, the lazy good-for-nothings won't do it; they just want to sit around and twiddle their thumbs and ask to be fed, and do nothing.'

Later on, as a result partly of mental health consultation in which I was involved, as well as of various other complicated factors, the style of the reception camps was radically changed. Newcomers were sent straight from the boat to small temporary encampments dotted about the countryside. They were housed as family units, at first only in canvas tents and later in crude tin huts. These were not as cool in summer or as water-tight in winter as the big army barrack huts, but they did protect the integrity of the family and its strength. Communal kitchens were not provided; each family had to fend for itself; and from the first they were given work to do, mostly difficult work, clearing rocky hillsides or draining swamps, but productive work which fostered their feelings of independence, and gave them immediately the feeling of being involved in a collaborative endeavour to build a homeland. Naturally, there have been many grumbles on the part of new immigrants who have been frightened by the isolation, the hard work, and the physical danger of exposure to marauding Arab attacks, but the former apathy and over-dependence have disappeared. On a recent visit to Israel I was very interested to find that there were still people living in the dirty, ramshackle remains of the big camps. The government had closed the camps down, but could do nothing with these inmates who had fallen into a completely dependent, apathetic state; and that is where they stay. Of course, the number of such die-hards is now quite small.

In Boston

Another example comes from Boston, Massachusetts; an example not, unfortunately, of successful action of the type that I have mentioned, but of the possibility for action. Across the street from the Whittier Street Health Center where I work in Roxbury, a rather poor suburb of Boston, there is a large new housing project. Nowadays it does not look very new; but about nine or ten years ago it was new and it looked new. Since it has been set up, there has been a steady drain on the budget of the City of Boston Health Department for the repair of broken windows in the Health Center building. The children used to spend much of their free time throwing stones through the windows; and it hardly ever happened that we would come to work in the morning without having to brush glass off the floor of our rooms before going near the window. There have been many other indications in the neighbourhood of an increase in destructive and delinquent acts by children of various ages. Now, the topic of juvenile delinquency is very complicated, and I do not wish to discuss it in the present context, but there are one or two factors in relation to the housing project which I believe are not insignificant.

First, we discovered when we looked at these housing projects that about 50 to 60 per cent of the families in them were broken families of one sort or another; that is, the mother had never had a husband, or he had left her, or it was a common-law marriage in uneasy equilibrium. The project population contains many other examples of social pathology. There appears to be a diffusion of culture from the unhealthy families to the previously healthy ones. A healthy family comes in and gets infected, as it were, like putting a new apple in a barrel where there are a lot of rotten ones. Some non-delinquent children after living a short time in the project join the delinquent gangs, the core of which appears to be made up of children from the disordered families.

There is nothing new in this, indeed it is quite usual; but if one asks how it happens that so high a proportion of the inhabitants of the housing projects are social deviants, one finds that to get into such a project a family has to be on a priority list, position on which depends upon a point system; and the point system is determined largely by the social need, so that the greater the social pathology, the more likely the family is to get to the top of the list. Moreover, in Boston as in other places, administrative difficulties are involved in getting into housing projects. No doubt

6

this does not apply in Denver or in Manchester, but in Boston in order to get into housing projects it is better if you have 'pull'. Once upon a time with the political boss system, and the ward system, the healthiest families were the ones that had the most 'pull'. They could get around and manipulate the politicians, but nowadays we have done away with that. Instead, the people who have the 'pull' are the social agencies. It is the social workers who apply pressure on behalf of their clients, and they can apply more pressure than an individual family can do on its own.

The reader may agree with me that it was a pity that a mental health worker was not present while that priority system was being worked out, in order to try to influence the administrators to plan some kind of balanced population for the project. Of course, research is needed to determine what is the critical proportion above which a housing project population cannot accept broken families without endangering its total morale. Given a housing project population, what proportion of disordered families can be introduced so that the disordered ones will be made healthier by the healthy ones, rather than the healthy ones be influenced by the unhealthy ones?

I have chosen these three examples to illustrate one type of Administrative Action for preventive psychiatry, the goal being the reduction of the incidence of stress situations, or the increase of the provision for the satisfaction of psychological needs. We have to realize, however, that we can never aim at removing all problems from the world, by ensuring that all people are satisfied. Suffering is going to be with us; illness and death are going to be with us for ever. We can, however, assist community leaders to arrange facilities so that people who are facing inevitable stress situations may be helped to solve their problems in a healthy way. There is a good deal of justification for thinking that the capacity for reality-based problem-solving is an excellent measure of the mental health of an individual or a group, and also for thinking that the way people handle any significant stress situation in a crisis will have far-reaching effects on their future mental health. Indeed, a good deal of the structure of society can be understood in terms of its purpose in supporting individual members in their solution of life's problems. All communities have specialized agencies and individuals who can be conceived of as 'caretaking agents', whose function it is to help people in various predicaments. These predicaments, such as birth, death, change of marital and other status, illness, change of occupation, and so on, are normally not conceived of by administrators as mental health crises; and, of course, primarily they are not. But community arrangements, such as agency structure and policy, will often affect in no small measure how individuals in these predicaments handle their problems and what the mental health consequences will be. How a given community deploys its limited caretaking resources may depend on all kinds of social and political forces. There is room in such planning for a mental health consultant who will advise on the effects of policies on the mental health of the population.

Prenatal and Postnatal Services

Let us take as an example the crisis of a woman having a baby. In the United States most communities provide prenatal clinics for checking the pregnant woman's physical state, obstetric hospitals for helping her give birth, and well-baby clinics for continued supervision of mother and infant. There is often a domiciliary nursing service such as a Visiting Nurse Association, which visits the home a few times during pregnancy and once or twice after delivery to supervise the woman's health. Many localities have a municipal health department which provides nurses who make one visit after the mother returns home from the lying-in hospital to check the baby's condition and to invite the mother to the well-baby clinic. But, in most localities, *all or most of these agencies operate separately, with little or no relationship with each other.* This may not be ideal policy from the point of view of the physical health of the mother and baby, but from the point of view of helping the mother handle the mental health crises of this crucial period it could not be worse.

A recent experiment conducted by the Harvard School of Public Health, the Boston Lying-In Hospital, and the Boston

Children's Hospital has shown the tremendous benefits to the developing mother-child and general family relationships of continuity of agency service throughout this period, based upon the fact that there is continuous support to the mother through the building up of a stable relationship, as well as the possibility, and this is very important, of predicting problems during pregnancy which can be nipped in the bud at that time or immediately afterwards, rather than allowed to run on until they become serious. I shall discuss this more fully in Chapters 3 and 4.

There is one other point that I should like to emphasize here. We found that one of the most difficult times for the mother is during the three to four weeks after she leaves the lying-in hospital. In most places this is a relative hiatus as far as agency service is concerned. The mother is usually expected to make her first visit to the well-baby clinic when the infant is about one month old. During that month she is left largely to her own resources unless she is lucky enough to have a supportive family around her. And I would point out that in a country like the United States the two sides of the family may come from different cultural backgrounds. This may be productive of much insecurity, because there may be the advocacy of two sets of differing ways of taking care of the baby. Furthermore, husband and wife may be of another culture from their parents (a subject I shall consider in Chapter 5) and so a three- or four-way conflict is possible in a significant proportion of cases. Everyone in the family, not to mention the neighbours, will be telling the mother something different.

A change of agency pattern suggested by the above work is intensive domiciliary supervision in certain cases during that particular period, and earlier contact with the well-baby clinic. This matter has been found to be of even more importance if there is something wrong with the baby, such as prematurity or a congenital abnormality, and these are not uncommon happenings. I have not been able to obtain from my paediatric and obstetric colleagues any certain estimate of the incidence of congenital abnormality, but the figure of 2 per cent is often quoted. Anyway, it is not a small figure, if all the degrees of congenital abnormali-

9

ties are included, so that we are here discussing a significant proportion of mothers who have babies. The baby may be very adequately cared for as regards his physical condition in the hospital; and in the case of prematurity many hospitals arrange for a nurse to visit the mother at home before the baby is discharged to make sure there are proper facilities to receive it. If she is a public health nurse who has plenty of time and a rather small case-load, she can in fact do more than just make a routine visit. Crippled children's services, however, do not come into action for many months or longer after the parents have had to deal *unaided* with the complicated emotional burden of adapting to the child's abnormality. How much time and wasted professional energy would be saved, not to mention avoidable unhappiness and personality distortions for family and child, if community leaders were to realize that a baby with a congenital abnormality is a situation requiring emergency agency attention concentrated and deployed at the critical period; that is, within the first two months after birth.

The type of caretaking personnel available to various agencies is also a matter with preventive psychiatric implications. If a community can afford a certain number of psychiatrists, psychiatric social workers, and public health mental health nurses, should these all be operating in remedial institutions, or should some of them be made available to work in agencies which deal, for example, with the ordinary woman having a baby? What are the needs for psychiatric assistance of an agency set up to help women with babies who are premature or have congenital abnormalities? Such questions point up one of the major difficulties facing a mental health specialist operating within a governmental or other executive group. He has to avoid taking on the role of an administrator himself, and to avoid giving advice based upon his own individual professional or political vested interests. I am not at all advocating government by psychiatrists! Moreover, present psychiatric knowledge about most of the practical issues which come up for administrative consideration is woefully inadequate. We just do not know the answers in a scientific way. The psychiatrist will rarely be in a position to press for some specific administrative action on sure grounds of scientific knowledge. His role is rather to put what knowledge he has at the disposal of the administrators and to avoid taking over their executive responsibility, either because of his own needs or because they try and talk him into doing so.

Now I wish to turn to the other main area, namely Personal Interaction.

PERSONAL INTERACTION

This category refers to preventive intervention that attempts to change the emotional forces in a person's environment or the way he solves his life's problems by direct interaction with that person or with the people immediately around him. It makes use more obviously of skills and insights which psychiatrists have developed in their clinical work with patients; and many of the techniques are clearly modifications of psychotherapeutic methods, which they resemble as much as they do educational techniques. It resembles Administrative Action in that the strategic goals relate to the planning for the reduction of emotional ill-health in the community as a whole. The greatest good for the greatest number implies a framework of action in which *economy of effort* is a prime consideration. It differs from Administrative Action in that the tactics in any instance are related to personal face-to-face contacts with individuals or small groups. So, the overall strategy relates to reduction of mental disorder in the community as a whole, but the way in which this goal is achieved is by dealing with individuals and small groups.

The goals are based upon a theory of aetiology which appears reasonable to us at the present time. As I said at the beginning of this chapter, we still do not know what are the causes of mental disorder, but we have some ideas; and I think it important to stress that preventive programmes do not have to be deferred until clear, scientifically validated proof of the aetiology of an illness is available. As a matter of fact, many of the advances in public health were made at a time when it was not known exactly what caused certain illnesses. Typhoid and smallpox were reduced before their exact causes were known; and at the present time there is still doubt about their causes, as advances are made into more and more abstruse areas of epidemiology and microbiology. It is not necessary to know all, but certain aspects of the aetiology must be fairly well understood. What is needed is a pretty good hunch, and the willingness to launch a programme before the hunch is validated.

Now this theory, or rather this collection of hunches, to which I am referring, holds that among the significant factors which will determine the mental health of an individual are those related to his emotional milieu, with special reference to the quality of interpersonal relationships obtaining between certain people in his immediate environment and himself. This is especially marked during childhood, and the influence of the parents' relationships upon the pattern of unfolding of personality development is well recognized. But it is also true in adult life, and this tends to be forgotten. In recent years we have come to place a considerable amount of emphasis on the idea that adequate gratification of the psychological needs of a person, and the degree to which he will be supported in times of stress, will depend, among other things, upon his relationships with his family, friends, and work groups. This will be an essential aspect of his life situation which will determine to a considerable degree whether he is or becomes mentally well or mentally ill. In other words, everyone, whether child or adult, has a certain range of basic prerequisites or needs (which will be discussed more fully in Chapter 5), and if these needs are satisfied he is likely to be mentally healthy. If they are unsatisfied, he is likely to move in a mentally unhealthy direction. Secondly, as he faces life's problems (see Chapter 2), one of the important factors in determining whether he deals with the problems in a healthy way, rather than in an unhealthy way, will be the influence of the people around him. What effect do they have upon him, and how do they help or hinder him at this time when he is wrestling with his difficulties?

I have already emphasized the multifactorial nature of the system, namely, that there are many factors involved, not just one or two; but a possible approach to a preventive programme might usefully be designed to improve interpersonal relationships or to remedy disordered ones, rather than to wait for the effect of these disordered relationships to lead to psychiatric pathology.

There is one other point that I wish to make in this connection, and that is that I am not talking now about an individual; I am talking about a community. If there is a higher proportion of disordered relationships in one community than in another, the likelihood is that there will eventually be a higher incidence of mental disorders in the first community than in the second community; although this will not determine the fate of any single individual in that community. As soon as focus is made on an individual, account must be taken of all kinds of idiosyncratic factors (some of which will be discussed in Chapter 2), which may outweigh the importance of these disordered relationships. That is to say, if a person is very robust constitutionally, resilient and strong, in perfect physical health, highly intelligent, and with stable control over his emotions, it does not matter too much whether he has a supportive family around him when he is in difficulty; he is going to get through all right. In considering him in particular, all these factors must be taken into account; but in considering a thousand people, these particular aspects will cancel out from one group to the other, and what then stands out is the importance of certain factors which operate on a community-wide scale in one instance, and on a community-wide scale in the other instance; and these are the kind of factors that I am talking about.

What can be said is that, in a community in which there are disordered relationships, it may be possible to intervene to improve interpersonal relationships or reduce the disordered relationships, and thus increase the number of mentally healthy people without waiting for these relationship disorders to foster mental illness. Now, stated like this, the goal is too broad for effective action.

Clinical experience shows that the scope of the problem can be narrowed down, because there exist in a community certain key individuals who are especially significant for a number of people by reason of their position in the role structure. When one of these key individuals has disordered relationships, he may affect the mental health of many people who are dependent upon him. He himself may or may not show overt signs of psychiatric illness, but he has an obvious noxious effect on the people around him. The analogy of the carrier of an infectious disease such as typhoid comes readily to mind. There appear to be 'Typhoid Marys' in the field of mental health, as there are in the field of physical health. The practical questions for a preventive programme in any community are to see whether such 'carriers' of mental ill-health can be detected; and, if so, whether their number is such that they can be dealt with; and if techniques can be worked out for improving their interpersonal relationships by methods which are economical enough in time and skilled manpower to allow of community coverage.

The Jerusalem Study

This was the kind of formulation we made in 1949 in Jerusalem; and since then we have developed it considerably. I should like to give a brief description of the practical steps we took there to implement such a plan.

We chose mothers of infants as our key people, based on the clinical experience that one mother with certain types of disordered relationship might have a pathogenic effect successively on several of her children. Moreover, our work in child guidance clinics had led us to suppose that we could define and identify the signs of disordered mother-child relationships which would mark any mother a 'carrier' or not; realizing, of course, that a particular mother would have idiosyncratic relationships with each of her children, but supposing that many mothers who showed a pathogenic relationship to one child would have a spread to others. (As a matter of fact in practice we find there are some mothers who single out one child in the family and have a pathogenic relationship only with that child, but there is also quite a large group of mothers who have a pathogenic relationship with all their children. Examination of their families shows that they exerted an unhealthy effect successively on the development of each of their children.) We then hunted in the communities for these 'carriers'. We narrowed our search down by focusing on well-baby clinics, where there is a high concentration of mothers of infants; and we developed rapid screening devices for scanning the total population of mothers in each clinic. We found that about 5 per cent of the mothers in the Jerusalem population were screened out as having undoubted or probable disordered relationships with their infants. We then worked out techniques for motivating these mothers to co-operate in the deeper investigations of their relationships. And where the original suspicion was found to be valid, we developed techniques of involving the mother in a treatment relationship. So we were able to screen the population and to get the mothers to co-operate.

The next step in the process was critical. Could we find methods of ameliorating the disordered relationships which would be *economical*? If the disorder were based on some neurosis of the mother, and all we had achieved by so much effort was a list of candidates for adult psychotherapy, we would not be much better off from a community point of view than if we had waited until the infant grew into a child with psychiatric symptoms and then treated these children as psychiatric patients. There would be some gain because we had one mother with a number of children, and we were treating one person instead of a number; but the gain would not be great enough.

We feel that one of the triumphs of this work in Jerusalem has been that we did manage to work out techniques of what we called 'unlinking' the child from the mother's intrapsychic disorders; that is, of improving the mother's relationships with this child and her other children, without having to become committed to undertaking the often major task of treating her core problems by lengthy methods of psychotherapy. We developed techniques of focused casework or psychotherapy, which concentrated on the *inter*personal problems of the mother, that is to say, the problems between the mother and the child, which in most cases did not encroach more than a minimum amount on her *intra*personal problems, the problems inside herself (I deal more fully with this particular principle in Chapters 4 and 7). We

15

found that in the majority of cases such techniques were possible, because the disorder in relationships involved only one segment of the range of emotional problems which had been crystallized in the personality pattern of the mother. In other words, we conceive of a personality as being a crystallization of successive patterns of successful or unsuccessful solutions to a multitude of problems that have occurred to that person all through his life up to that time. We discovered that many cases of disordered mother-child relationships represented a partial solution of some of the woman's past problems. And in many of the cases, the problems which were solved by having the disordered relationship with the child were peripheral to the central problems which had been solved in the development of the mother's personality. So we did not have to go into the main personality problems; we just dealt with one part at the edge.

The impressions gained in this study were that it is certainly practical to go into a community and to identify a major proportion of those mothers who have pathogenic relationships with their infants, and it is possible to think in practical terms of deploying sufficient skilled staff to remedy these disorders. A point I shall stress continually throughout this book is that the goal is to achieve coverage of all the problems in the community, and not deal with just 1 per cent of them; this is the usual percentage dealt with by a typical remedial psychiatric institution like a child guidance clinic, which in a community of 500,000 will have a case-load of, say, 250 – a drop in the ocean. If the aim is a therapeutic approach and high-quality work with a small number of patients, this is admirable; but if we are concerned with prevention and with reducing the incidence of cases of mental disorder in a community, we cannot be satisfied with that. We have constantly to bear in mind that we have to develop a programme which is going to deal with the community as a whole. Now, the average number of sessions per case in the present technique was about eight or ten. Group techniques could probably be developed to make such a plan even more practical from a community point of view. But both individual and group techniques demand a staff of experienced and highly trained psychiatric workers, which is not likely to be available except in a few privileged communities.

Moreover, since 1949, we have become rather more sophisticated about analysing the field of forces in a person's emotional milieu; and we can no longer think without discomfort of isolating mother-child relationships in as static a way as we did then. For instance, we were impressed in Jerusalem by the fact that in certain cases we benefited the mother-child relationship, and the follow-up investigation showed a subsequent, and maybe a consequent, disturbance of wife-husband relationship, or some other subtle alteration in the field of forces in the family. Even for the original infant, when he had developed past the stage of almost complete dependence on his mother, the change in family equilibrium that resulted from the original unlinking manoeuvre was sometimes as productive of psychiatric disturbance as the original situation would have been. In other words, if the woman was prevented from solving those particular problems through the disordered relationship with her child, she may have started solving them by having a disordered relationship with her husband, or by altering her way of handling affairs in the family, so that the previous equilibrium of the rest of the family became disturbed, and the end result may have been worse than the first one, even though, during the period of his infancy, her relationship with her child might have been 'healthy'.

Another relevant consideration is the idea that we might track down the factors that actually lead to disordered mother-child relationships. That is to say, instead of working on the disordered mother-child relationships themselves, we might deal with the forces that produce them; and this might be easier than the highly skilled job of segmental casework. It might be so easy that it could be entrusted to public health workers who have had no lengthy psychiatric training. This hope was spurred on by the discovery that certain traumatic events during pregnancy, such as a failed attempt at abortion, or the death or injury of another child, often led to especially pathogenic types of disorders of the future mother-child relationship.

The unhealthy development in such cases can often be nipped

in the bud fairly easily by public health nurses, by paediatricians, by obstetricians, or by hospital nurses, who are alerted to the special mental health significance of certain traumatic events, and equipped with minor mental health first-aid techniques, such as methods of reducing excessive conscious or preconscious guilt.

Such thinking, then, highlighted the importance of certain experiences in Jerusalem, and similar experiences in Boston, where my colleague Erich Lindemann had been working on the manifestations of the bereavement process in adults, and its relationship to the subsequent development of various psychiatric disorders. I describe this work in Chapters 2 and 8, but I wish to mention here that the concept that emerged was one that has been familiar to lay people, and to novelists and dramatists, for centuries, but until now has received scant attention from psychiatrists : namely, the importance of periods of *crisis* in determining individual and group development.

Crisis

Such a crisis is provoked when a person faces an obstacle to important life goals that is, for a time, insurmountable through the utilization of customary methods of problem-solving. A period of disorganization ensues, a period of upset, during which many different abortive attempts at solution are made. Eventually some kind of adaptation is achieved, which may or may not be in the best interests of that person and his fellows. The important point for the development of our present theme is that disturbances of interpersonal relationships between mothers and children, and also within the total field of forces in a family, can often be seen clinically to originate during a certain crisis period, or subsequent to a certain crisis period; and can be conceived of as one type of maladaptive solution of the crisis problem – a vicarious solution by projection and displacement at the emotional expense of someone within the family orbit.

In an oversimplified way, we can say that the crisis was resolved by means of the development of the disordered relationship. I hinted at this when I referred to a woman who had a variety of problems and, after the arrival of a baby, solved some of her problems by relating to the baby in a certain distorted way. I discuss such cases in detail in Chapters 3 and 6, but for the present purpose it is enough to suppose that she had a problem with her sister with which she was not able to deal. Then along comes the baby, and the baby turns out to be a girl; and now she reacts to the baby as though the baby were her sister. Or she had an emotional problem in relation to her father, who died when she was pregnant, and she could not deal with his death; she could not adapt to it by doing her grief-work properly, which I discuss in Chapters 2 and 8. When the baby is born she unconsciously invests the child with the characteristics of her father. It often happens that she names it after her father, and she deals with it as though her father continues to live through this child. This then disturbs her relationship with the child, so that she can no longer see her child in its own right but sees instead a father-figure there. Some readers may think it strange for a woman to react to a little infant as though it were her father, but a review of clinical experience would show that these things are not so very unusual.

Such considerations have led to a research project at present being conducted at the Harvard School of Public Health Family Guidance Center at Whittier Street, about which I am going to report in more detail in Chapter 5. A number of categories of commonly occurring stress have been chosen, such as the birth of a premature baby, or the birth of a baby with a congenital abnormality, or a diagnosis of tuberculosis in a family member. Families who are in crisis as a result of these problems are then studied with the intention of describing the range of adaptive and maladaptive responses.

The hope is that it will be possible to separate at one end of the spectrum those families who have found a solution of the crisis problem by developing disordered relationships. It is further hoped that, in the same way that Lindemann, by his study of normal grief in bereavement, can now help to steer back on to the adaptive path those bereaved persons who show signs of deviating, the present study will equip us with specific information to help families in crises. In other words, if we know how families in one of these crises deal with the crisis problem in a healthy way, and if we can spot those who are showing signs of not dealing with it in this way, our knowledge of the healthy ways of dealing with crises will allow us to intervene and to steer the latter families on to the healthy path. What is very important is that this can be done *without having to know why it is that the unhealthy families were on the unhealthy path*. This is the crux of the matter. It is not necessary to analyse the original deep reasons inside the personalities of these people, which made it difficult for them to handle the problem in a healthy way. As long as it can be ensured that they do handle it in a healthy way when they are helped, then the outcome will be benign.

I would emphasize that such techniques are of a superficial variety; they require little time and not too much training, since they handle mainly preconscious mechanisms. They do not delve into the dynamics of the unconscious personality. In other words, they would be available for widespread use in the health setting, and such a service would make use of psychiatric personnel mainly in a consultative or advisory role. This leads me on to a consideration of possibly the most important type of preventive psychiatric activity, which comes under the heading of Personal Interaction, namely mental health consultation.

Mental Health Consultation

In my booklet *Concepts of Mental Health and Consultation* (Caplan, 1959) I have gone into considerable detail about mental health consultation. Some of it is relevant to work in nursing; some of it is focused on the needs of social workers in a public health setting.

I have referred above to key people who exert a potent effect upon the mental health of a number of other individuals. When I first discussed this concept I had in mind blood relations, close friends, or people occupying special roles in a person's work or recreation group; and it became rapidly obvious that in a community there existed a network of institutional roles which fitted into this category, namely people like nurses, doctors, clergymen, teachers, policemen, and so on. These are the caretaking agents of the community. At particular times they are certainly key people in affecting the mental health of many others. It is significant that these particular times are usually times of crisis for their clients. The school-teacher, for example, is of importance to the educational progress of her students. To some extent she is important to their mental health, according to the general type of interpersonal relationships she manifests, and the consequent emotional atmosphere she builds up in her classroom. But her importance as a factor in the emotional life of some particular student suddenly increases tremendously when that student is faced by a crisis problem. At that time the supportive or unhelpful activities of the teacher may be instrumental in tipping the child towards or away from a healthy adaptive solution of his life's problem. The same situation can be seen to hold with clergymen, and even more so with nurses and doctors. The quality of care which these people are able to deliver, when an individual or a family is in crisis, may be a crucial factor in determining the outcome as far as the future mental health of their client is concerned.

Each one of these professional caretaking groups has its own sub-culture, its own traditional ways of perceiving its client's problems and of handling them. They may be thought of in terms of having what I have called a 'professional persona', a professional personality, a fairly standardized range of ways of handling their professional problems including the usual human reactions of their clients who are in crisis. This range is usually flexible and allows for individual variation according to the idiosyncratic personality structure of the individual professional worker. For instance, not all nurses handle the same problem in the same way, and yet they may all be handling it efficiently from a nursing point of view.

Changing Professional Roles

Two points are of interest in this connection. First, are the traditional ways of helping people, in line with the professional persona, effective from a mental health point of view? It must be realized that the primary purpose of the professional persona is

21

not the pursuit of mental health, but the pursuit of the primary goal of that profession – teaching, doctoring, nursing, and so on. If the traditional ways are not effective for mental health, can we work out ways of making them more effective, ways which are compatible with the primary goals and the general framework of that profession? It is no good trying to make nurses into psychiatrists. Even if we succeeded, we would then need to look for people to train as nurses. A nurse has to cover a certain ground in which she is a specialist, and no other profession deals with those problems in that way. The ways that nurses have developed in dealing with these problems have over the years proved to be the best which fit in with the goals and traditions of nursing. If the nurse's role is altered so that she begins to work like a psychologist or a psychiatrist or a social worker, it may result in her being no good as a nurse. And we do need to have nurses!

The role of the nurse. I have been interested in the last few years in the problems of nursing in general hospitals, and I have discovered that the professional persona of the general hospital nurse is in flux; she is being changed; and in many hospitals she has already been changed a good deal. Rapidly advancing technology in medicine and surgery means that patients in a good general hospital are dealt with very differently nowadays from what they were fifteen years ago. There are all kinds of abstruse machines in operation on the wards. A patient does not just lie in a bed, he is attached to all kinds of tubes, to all kinds of electrical and mechanical gadgets around him; he is also having injections of all kinds of new drugs. And the person dealing with all this is the general hospital nurse. In addition, the whole rate of turnover in the hospital has altered because of the changed technology, and because of the increasing age of the general hospital population. The numbers and types of cases being dealt with are different from in the past, and this leads to different types of hospital administration. For instance, in one general hospital that I know, the hospital is still run as though the daytime is the time when the hospital operates normally; and at night there is a skeleton staff because at night it is supposed that the hospital just ticks over; but investigation reveals that there are almost as many surgical operations at night as there are during the day, and that there are as many ward rounds by residents after 11.0 p.m. as before 11.0 p.m. The whole pattern has altered. The amount of administrative detail has increased enormously, and the nurse is responsible for much of this. It is very nice that she is; but the only thing is that the nurse in the general hospital has now become quite a different professional person from what she was before; and the question is: 'Who does the bedside nursing?' And so it appears that there is now a hiatus; there is a nursing role that nurses used to do; nurses are now doing something else, and people are needed to train to act as bedside nurses. In many hospitals practical nurses and nurses' aids are doing the bedside nursing, and the registered nurses have become technological or administrative assistants. This may be good, bad, or indifferent, but it is a significant change; and I think that whenever new concepts and roles are introduced into any profession, great care must be taken to safeguard its traditional roles.

What is needed from the point of view of planning mental health programmes is a study of what the range of operations is in the different professions plus a good deal more research along Whittier Street lines to provide specific information about the most helpful behaviour by caretaking agents during crisis periods. This is one aspect of the problem.

Personality Factors and Professional Role

The second aspect of the problem is how do individual personality factors interfere with the professional persona, and what can be done to prevent either generalized disorders of interpersonal functioning, or specific upsets in the caretaking agent, from interfering with his capacity to help his clients in crisis?

To illustrate this point let me quote two familiar examples. A public health nurse encounters special difficulty whenever she deals with the problems of an old man living on his own. In such cases she usually becomes emotionally involved and upset and is unable to operate with her customary effectiveness. If we were to investigate her background, we would probably find that in the past in her own private life she had had some traumatic experience in relation to an aged relative. Maybe when she was a child she was an impotent bystander while a beloved grand-father was being rejected by the other members of her family. At that time she could not understand the issues involved and was herself unable to interfere in the affair. She may have repressed all memory of this sad experience, but her feelings of misery and guilt are likely to be stimulated over and over again whenever she comes in contact with an old man in similar circumstances.

Another example is the young nurse who is at present in con-flict over the question of marriage, or the nurse who has recently married and is worried lest she has become pregnant at a time when she is trying to earn money in order to help her young husband through university. Such a nurse is not unlikely to have some difficulty in handling the problems of a patient in similar circumstances. Strangely enough, she may not always see the obvious link between her own problems and those of her patient. All she may be aware of is that she is having difficulty in dealing with the case. Someone else looking at her would say, 'Of course one can't expect you to be able to handle a case like this at the present time because you are so upset about this topic yourself.' As a matter of fact, if this was said to her, it probably would not do her much good. The reason for this is that most of us try to keep our private life and our professional work separate. We all know that not only our patients but we ourselves are human beings with emotional problems, but the essence of professional functioning is to keep our own private problems out of the work field. In our professional training we develop a so-called 'profes-sional armour', a professional distance between ourselves and our patients. An essential difference between an amateur and a professional is that the professional has this distance, and deals objectively rather than subjectively with the problems of his clients.

It is rather important to maintain this 'professional armour' intact, because, although it might be helpful in a particular case to develop insight into the personal source of our professional difficulties, once this armour has been punctured we shall feel more vulnerable in such situations in the future, because we shall always be worrying lest our personal problems should once again interfere with our work.

If nurses, paediatricians, obstetricians, and general practitioners are to be expected to deal with the mental health problems of their patients, which are of so universal a nature that not infrequently they will be dealing with problems about which they themselves have some personal sensitivity, how can this problem be handled? How can we handle the fact that the caretaking agents are apt to be stimulated by the crises of their clients?

Consultation with School-teachers

One way which has been developed in order to try to handle this problem is what has been called mental health consultation. This method has been worked out during the past ten years. It was developed originally for work with school-teachers, but in more recent years it has been extended to helping public health nurses, paediatricians, probation officers, clergymen, and other professional workers handle the mental health problems of their clients. In its traditional method of operation the mental health specialist goes around from school to school and offers to discuss with the school-teachers any of their students with emotional difficulties with whom they are having some trouble. The causes of the difficulty a school-teacher may be having in managing the mental health complications of a student can usually be divided into three categories.

In many cases these difficulties are based upon the fact that the teacher has an inadequate understanding of psychological matters in general and of the particular factors involved in the present case. The mental health consultant's task is then to help her, through a discussion of this case, to understand more fully what is going on in this child and in his family, so that the teacher may develop a deeper insight into the particular situation. We have found that on the basis of this increased insight the teacher is usually able to handle the case successfully on her own.

The second category of cases relates to a situation where the teacher's difficulty is not due to any lack of insight and understanding into the causation of the child's difficulty, but to the fact that she does not know what course of action to take. The teacher may never have met a case like this before, or her school may not have the facilities to handle such cases, or she may not know that there exist appropriate facilities in the community to handle such a case, or she may know about the existence of specialist resources but have no channels of communication in order to refer the child and his family to such an agency. It is then the task of the consultant to help the teacher review the various possibilities of action in order to handle the problem, or to help her explore the avenues along which specialist help may be obtained for the child.

The third type of situation is the one to which I have previously referred, where the human problems of the teacher interfere with her handling of the case. In this situation it is the task of the consultant to assess what particular aspect of the case is especially difficult for the teacher because of her human sensitivities, and to give her focused support and help in overcoming this particular difficulty in the child. The consultant, as it were, lends his own strength to the teacher in helping the child in an area where the teacher on her own would be incapacitated. In a successful case, when the teacher with the assistance of the consultant is able to help the student with his current life problem, this has a unique significance to her. She now feels less tense in regard to this particular topic than she did before, and an area of her professional functioning that in the past had been a source of special difficulty may now become an area in which she is able to operate with her customary effectiveness.

It is important to emphasize that this whole process is carried out without the consultant ever attempting to find out the source of the consultee's difficulty in her private life situation. The issue of the consultee's personal problems is never raised explicitly in the consultation discussion. It is in fact not necessary for the consultant to know exactly what it is in the private life of the consultee which has made her sensitive in this special area. All he has to know is that there is something which is causing her to have some difficulties in regard to some particular aspect of the case, so that he can handle this aspect with special sensitivity to the feelings of the consultee, and make directed efforts to be helpful in relation to this special theme. Since the consultee's personal problems are never discussed, this differentiates the consultation process clearly from psychotherapy or casework. The consultee is always treated with respect as a professional colleague, and is never treated as a patient or client. It is taken for granted that everyone is entitled to have his own private personal problems. In the work field all that interests us is that the work should be carried out effectively, and the details of our private problems are not relevant to consultation discussions.

It takes a fair degree of skill for the mental health consultant to be able to handle these sensitive areas in such a way as to avoid infringing on the privacy of the consultee, but we have been able to train quite a number of people to do this kind of work in the past seven or eight years. In the Commonwealth of Massachusetts at the present time we have about fifty trained mental health consultants at work, and a similar programme is also being set up in the State of California.

In these programmes a small number of highly trained mental health specialists have access to a large number of caretaking agents – teachers, physicians, nurses, and so on – and these care-taking agents are helped to improve their attention to the mental health dimension of their routine everyday work.

THE PROBLEM OF MOTIVATION

Before concluding this chapter, it seems advisable to focus specifically on the problem of motivation in preventive psychiatry. This raises the question of one essential difference between preventive work and therapeutic work. In therapeutic work you can rely upon a fairly high degree of motivation in your patient. The patient has a pain and comes to you and says, 'Please cure me of my pain.' Because he feels the pain and wants you to cure him he will be willing to put up with all kinds of inconvenience. He will be willing to undress, to allow you to stick needles into him, and to allow you to heap all kinds of indignities upon him. But in preventive work you are dealing with a person who is not in pain, and may not be aware that there is any risk of ever getting a pain. This important stimulus to motivation to involve himself with you in your professional endeavours is therefore missing, and the arousal of this motivation becomes a difficult technical issue.

Experience shows that, although this problem is not easy, it can be dealt with by a variety of techniques, one or two of which I shall briefly mention. The main approach is to stimulate the arousal of a meaningful emotional relationship between the person and yourself. On the basis of this emotional link he may be willing to involve himself in your professional endeavours. He will do this in the first instance because he likes you and because he feels that you are interested in his life. The main method of fostering such a relationship is to present yourself as an understanding person who wishes to be helpful, and at the same time to identify and remedy the person's negative feelings towards you as they arise. For instance, you may inadvertently do something to cause him some feeling of pain or discomfort. However careful we are we very often stand on people's toes, as it were. In dealing with another person of whose idiosyncrasies we are unaware we must be very careful about this. We have, therefore, to keep a sensitive watch on the other person's behaviour, and if we find that we are standing on his toe we must take our foot off and immediately apologize.

Another common difficulty which interferes with the building up of a positive relationship is the feeling of the other person that you are looking down upon him. This is often based upon his feeling guilty about something. If this feeling of guilt is aroused during your conversation with him and you do nothing about it he will probably not come back to see you a second time. It is therefore important always to be on the lookout for feelings of guilt in an interviewee and to take immediate action in order to reduce them.

Let us take as an example a woman who has attempted abortion. From the way she speaks you may suspect that she has tried to terminate her pregnancy by taking pills, or by running up and down stairs, or by taking hot baths, or by horse-riding, or by some other means. It may be obvious that she is keeping all this a secret. Nevertheless, from her statements and from her demeanour you may be able to suspect something of the sort. It is very important to realize that she may guess that you suspect. If, however, you make no reference to your suspicion she is going to think, 'He suspects my guilty secret and he thinks that I am some kind of monster. I had better escape from him.' In these circumstances the important point is to let the woman know that you realize what she has done and that despite this you do not think that she is a monster. At the same time it would be very silly indeed to attempt to reduce her guilt by making her believe that you do not feel that she has done anything wrong. Many people would consider that a woman who has attempted to abort herself has done something which is against her religion and which is also probably against our religion, whatever that may be. We would feel that she has done something which in our culture is regarded as sinful, and she should feel guilty about it.

Guilt is, after all, a very useful feeling from a social point of view. Nobody becomes socialized solely on the basis of expectations of receiving love. Socialization is also based on expectations of punishment.

It would be quite wrong to give the woman the impression that you think abortion is perfectly all right. Paradoxically, if you do this you are likely to make her feel more guilty, and to make her feel that you yourself are an evil person, since you appear to condone evil. She will probably try to escape from you as quickly as possible, because she is likely to feel that she has already enough evil inside herself without being associated with a devil like you.

What needs to be done in such a case is to let the woman know that you have known many people who have done what she has done. Attempting abortion is a wrong thing to do and a feeling of guilt is a natural consequence. In her religion there are undoubtedly ways of dealing with feelings of guilt, but the trouble with her is that her feelings of guilt are out of all proportion to what should be expected from someone who has attempted abortion. This woman's trouble is that she feels that she is entirely bad and that she is a monster; but in fact she is an ordinary woman who gave way in a moment of weakness and attempted to find some desperate way out of her predicament. So what you have to try to communicate to her, in order to reduce her guilt to normal proportions, is that you understand her predicament, and although you know or guess that she did this particular wrong thing, you do not because of this consider her to be outside the pale of mankind, you do not rule her out of God's universe, you do not consign her to everlasting hell, and in fact you are prepared to go on talking with her in a friendly manner and to do whatever you can to help her. Conveying this information may allow her sufficient freedom in her relationship with you to discuss very frankly what she has done, and it may then be possible to support her in developing a more balanced appraisal of her actions and of herself as a person.

If in your conversation with your interviewee you are able to avoid inflicting pain, if you can reduce guilt, if you treat the person with respect, and if you offer yourself as a helping and supporting person, then your interviewee is likely to develop a positive and trusting relationship to you. On the basis of this you may then be able to say, 'Let us talk once or twice about the situation in which you find yourself, and it may be that I can be of some assistance to you.'

SUMMARY

To summarize, I have discussed the provision of services for a community programme of primary prevention in psychiatry which are aimed at: (*a*) the reduction of the occurrence of psychological stress in a community, and the increased provision for satisfying the psychological needs of individuals; and (*b*) help with problem-solving for individuals facing crisis situations, so that they may emerge from the crisis period with improved potential for mental health.

These services may be provided by modifying the behaviour of large sections of the population through governmental action, and also by preventive intervention which is focused upon individuals through methods based upon face-to-face contact. The latter category includes:

(*a*) *Direct Intervention* focused on the individual and his emotionally meaningful milieu during crisis.

(*b*) *Indirect Intervention* through the amelioration of disturbed interpersonal relationships focusing upon the individual which would have the effect of interfering with the long-term satisfaction of his psychological needs.

(*c*) *Indirect Intervention* by the provision of mental health consultation to the community caretaking agents whose role brings them into contact with the individual during his period of crisis.

REFERENCE

CAPLAN, GERALD (1959). *Concepts of Mental Health and Consultation*. Washington, D.C.: Children's Bureau Publication No. 373.

CHAPTER 2

Relevant Aspects of Ego Psychology
and their Relation to Preventive Intervention

I SHALL now take up some of the aspects of individual psychology which have a bearing on themes developed later in this book. I am going to discuss some of the newest ideas in the field, rather than cover ground already familiar. This field of individual psychology and personality theory is not in a static condition. Though there is a great deal we do not know, there is a great deal of thinking towards theoretical formulations which get closer to the facts than we have been able to manage in the past.

I am going to start from the assumption that you all know, more or less, the kind of things that were in the booklet *Concepts of Mental Health and Consultation* (1959). There are four technical terms that I shall employ, and I think it may be just as well for me very rapidly to review them. They are Ego, Superego, Ego Ideal, and Id.

These concepts are part of a structural theory of the personality. One can think of personality in terms of structure. Of course, this is a pure conceptualization because it does not really have a structure. There is no such thing as a 'thing' called personality. However, for descriptive purposes psychologists have found it useful to conceptualize the essence of human behaviour by thinking in terms of structure and function.

Personality from the structural point of view, according to one school of thought to which I subscribe, can be divided up into a number of parts. First, a large part, the most primitive, with which one is born, which is called the *Id*. It was given that name because it is an incoherent primitive aspect of personality. This is the irrational aspect. It is the repository of the instinctual forces, the biological drives.

The part to which I shall devote the greater part of this chapter is the *Ego*, the 'I', the essential core of the personality. There is also the *Superego*, which is really part of the ego, although it is described as a separate structure. It includes the conscience, the part which tells us what not to do, which is an internalization during growth and development of the values of our family primarily, and of our society generally.

Another internalized aspect of the ego is called the *Ego Ideal*. This is the part of the personality which tells us what to do, what to strive for, what our goals are, what our ideals are. The ego ideal also represents the internalized values of our family and of our society, and gives us some concept of our role in life. This moulds our actions by affirming our goals. The superego is the internalized value system which tells us what not to do. The ego itself is the main planning and perceiving, operating and controlling part of the personality.

The division of mental functioning into conscious and unconscious aspects is well known. We have realized for many years that much of our thinking goes on below the level of consciousness, and it is important to know that there is an unconscious aspect of the ego, an unconscious aspect of the superego, and an unconscious aspect of the ego ideal. The level of conscious and unconscious cuts across all three; and, of course, the id is totally unconscious.

THE EGO AND ITS FUNCTIONS

1. *Cognition.* The ego is the main executive aspect of the personality and its functions include first of all cognition – seeing, hearing, knowing, receiving stimuli from the outside world as well as from the inside world of the rest of the personality. If you think of yourself, you not only know what is going on in the outside world, but you also know what is going on inside you. You may

if you wish become conscious to a certain degree of your physical being and also of the state of the rest of your personality.

2. *Selection and integration.* The second function of the ego part of the personality is selecting and integrating these stimuli, once they have been recorded. They are integrated with records of past stimuli, with memory; and they are thus invested with meaning. The ego is not purely a mechanical device for recording stimuli. The stimuli come into the ego, and the ego then performs a very complex set of operations (which have actually been mimicked in various calculating machines, the mechanical brains) whereby the message which comes in is given meaning by virtue of the fact that it is connected with all kinds of other messages that have been received in the past. The first function is called perception, the second function is called, by some people, apperception.

3. *Planning.* The third function of the ego is planning for problem-solving. The messages come in; they are invested with meaning. The ego is then faced by a situation that has meaning and that presents it with a problem. The whole complicated set of operations involving planning and deciding what one ought to do about the problem forms an important part of ego-functioning.

4. *Control.* The fourth function of the ego is control – control of motility and control of impulse. This is the function which is involved with the implementation of a plan. In planning, we first of all see what the problem is, then we have to analyse it, and then we have to do something about it. The ego is conceptualized as having the function of executing the plan.

5. *Synthesis.* The fifth aspect of ego-functioning is synthesis. The ego is the executive aspect of personality which produces an equilibrium among the various forces that impinge upon it. Upon the ego impinge pressures and demands from the superego, from the ego ideal, and from the id. From the superego the message is, 'You must not do this'; from the ego ideal, 'You have to do that'; from the id, there are demands for satisfaction of the primitive impulses, the sexual, the aggressive, and the various physical

appetites. From the external world come the demands and challenges of the physical and social reality. The person has to be in equilibrium not only with the forces inside but with the forces outside himself. You do certain things or do not do other things, not only because there is something inside you that says do not do this or do that, but also because of the pressure and the support of the people around you, and of the physical reality of your environment.

Synthesis is one of the most interesting aspects of the ego, because what you see in a personality is a certain identity, a certain cohesiveness, and a certain predictability. If you get to know someone, you may be able to guess that he is going to behave in a certain way under certain conditions; and you can expect he will behave in a consistent way.

The consistency is a very special part of ego-functioning. It is the aspect of the synthesizing function which produces the identity of the person. Identity is something that can be perceived by others and of which also one has a sense oneself. One aspect of this synthesis, together with the perceptive and cognitive functions of the ego, is that one is aware of one's own identity. Where that awareness is disturbed we get a very interesting and painful disturbance of the personality.

6. *Object relations.* The last function of the ego that I shall describe is what is known in technical parlance as 'object relations', meaning relationships with other people. Other people, in psychoanalytic psychology, are given this rather unfortunate term of 'objects'. By object relations is meant the relationships of the person with other human beings in the world; but not only with human beings, and I think that is why we use the term 'objects', since one can have relationships with animals, and also with inanimate things, such as automobiles. Many of us have relationships with our car, sometimes of an intimate nature. We get very attached to it and we may become upset if someone else drives it; we may feel it does not run quite the same afterwards. When we have to sell it we have a period of mourning as though we have lost a loved object.

So much for a brief introduction to ego psychology. In addition I wish to mention that the ego in its relationships to the superego, ego ideal, the pressures of reality, and the forces from the id, can be thought of as defending itself against these various forces impinging upon it, and making use of some of the energy of the forces for its own purposes. It develops what are called 'defence mechanisms' to accomplish this. Anna Freud's book *The Ego and the Mechanisms of Defence* (1937) is as good a primer on this aspect of ego psychology as I know.

ASPECTS OF MENTAL HEALTH

I want to continue by discussing some aspects of mental health. Mental health as a concept is a very fuzzy one and it is really not a useful scientific concept at all, any more than physical health is, but used in quite a loose way, it is valuable as a focal concept. If you wish to assess the status of a person's mental health, you have obviously to take into account, and this is what makes it so fuzzy, the culture in which he is living, and the values of the culture and of yourself, as a person who is assessing his mental health. For instance, someone in the Army who wants to select a mentally healthy paratrooper is going to use a quite different set of values to assess his mental health from those applied by a member of a selection committee appointing a professor of nursing. The different context and the different kinds of people involved in doing the selecting will produce quite different results. Someone who is a mentally healthy professor of nursing would not look at all like a mentally healthy paratrooper – at least, I hope not.

Among the most important aspects of mental health is the state of the ego. What has to be assessed is the quality of the ego structure, and the stage of its development, or what is called the maturity of the ego. We realize that personalities develop, even possibly from before birth, but certainly during life; and they continue developing throughout life. They do not stop developing at the age of five or six, as some people used to think. Therefore, if you wish to assess a person's personality, one of the criteria you may use is the stage of his development.

In trying to assess the state of the ego of a person, there are three main areas at which you might look.

1. *Reaction to Stress*

First of all, you would look at the capacity of this person to withstand frustration and to tolerate anxiety and depression. According to latest ideas, these are the two principle reactions of the ego to difficulties; so if you want to assess the capacity of the ego, one of the ways is to see how it stands up to stress. You see how resilient it is, how flexible, how much it will bend, and under what conditions it breaks. What is being assessed is the degree of control of the ego in maintaining its equilibrium in the face of different pressures.

2. *Problem-solving*

The second area you would look at concerns the way this person solves his problems. In what degree is his solution of problems reality based when he is faced by a difficulty? If he perceives a threat or a challenge from outside, does he react to it in such a way that he is effective in the world of reality; or, on the other side of the scale, does he solve his problems through fantasy and magic, that is to say, by internal, intrapsychic manipulations? The ego has control of what is going on inside to some extent, and by playing a few little tricks a person can pretend that he has dealt with the problem in the outside world, despite the fact that he has not dealt with it at all. There are a variety of ways of pretending.

Another way of dealing with problems is by passive surrender or disintegration, which is called alienation. The person just cuts himself off from the whole world and goes back to his primitive non-thinking state. I suppose the paradigm of this is to become unconscious, in which case the person cuts off everything, and just lies there unfeeling. That is one way of dealing with the problem, though not a very effective one. The other way of dealing with it, short of complete unconsciousness, is complete or partial disintegration of personality functioning, which is called a psychosis. Fifty or sixty years ago psychiatrists were called alienists, because they dealt with alienated people, people who became strangers to the world of reality. This was quite a good term.

3. *Adjustments to Reality*

The third area of ego function that you would try to assess would be to see how far the person has achieved a happy balance between, on the one hand, gratification of his needs and instincts and impulses and, on the other hand, sacrifice of the gratification of these needs to the demands of reality, whether material reality, physical reality, or social reality. You would look to see, on the occasions when he does not gratify his impulses, to what extent this sacrifice is rendered palatable by abstract thinking and by fantasies of future pleasures, or by the satisfaction of 'higher social values'. This is an internal manipulation by the ego which is very much culturally based, and varies from one socio-economic class to another. In the U.S.A. this internal manipulation is commonest in middle-class people. It is a device that enables people to remain relatively happy and contented and in a stable state without increase of tension in a situation where they cannot currently gratify certain impulses. The other technique which is used is to rely on the fact that one is satisfying not the id, but the superego and ego ideal. We feel satisfaction from knowing we are living a good life, and we know that the person who lives a good life does not steal or does not go sleeping with someone else's wife, and so on.

During the whole of our lives, the ego is developing a repertoire of coping techniques in situations of difficulty. This repertoire of techniques, of ways of handling difficulty, both external and internal, is accumulated partly by the experience of having faced difficulties, having gone through crises, and having overcome them in certain novel ways. These ways then become part of the coping repertoire, and the repertoire is thus enriched. It may be enriched in a negative way, but in any case it is added to. The repertoire of coping methods is also added to by education. We are taught explicitly or implicitly how to deal with problem situations. The third way in which the repertoire is added to is through identification with other people who are using certain coping mechanisms. That is to say, one is on intimate terms with some other person who acts as a model; and then either consciously or unconsciously one copies the way the other person sees problems and deals with them. He can be described as a 'role model'. We incorporate the coping methods used by these other people. These are not just any other people, but important other people, like mothers and fathers, older brothers, teachers, and ministers.

What are the various situations of difficulty which precipitate crises? This relates to some of the questions that were raised in Chapter 1. I discussed certain hazardous circumstances, and said that these might produce a crisis in some people and not in others. Situations of difficulty can be broadly divided into two types. One type is a threat involving the danger of the loss of an object, or of a source of satisfaction of needs, or a threat to the integrity of one's body. In other words, there is a threat that you might lose something or someone you love. You might lose the opportunity to gratify yourself, or you might lose your arm or your leg or your life. From a certain point of view, I suppose, if you starve, you are losing integrity; there is the loss of the wherewithal to maintain physical existence at a satisfactory level. That is one kind of difficulty. The other kind of difficulty is not the threat of loss, but the loss itself, as when you actually lose an object, a person whom you love, a source of gratification; or when you lose your integrity and become damaged, injured. A variation on this is not an actual loss but an obstacle which stands in your way, which you have to overcome in order to achieve the object of gratification or your integrity.

Now the person that we are thinking about, when he faces either a threat of loss or loss itself, has a certain repertoire of responses, of ways of dealing with the situation. The type of repertoire will determine the type of person he is. If you talk about personality type, from one important aspect you are really talking about this. The other point which becomes obvious, from what I have said, is that if you distinguish between people with richer personalities and people with poorer personalities, what you may be implying is that the former have a larger variety of ways of handling situations so that they can handle more situations of difficulty in rather flexible ways. The more constricted or impoverished persons, on the other hand, are those who can operate only under certain quite fixed sets of conditions. If they are taken outside those limits, they will not have the social and psychological skills to handle the situation.

You can think of personality development as being in certain respects the enriching of the repertoire of social and other coping responses.

Now I want to link up with what we were talking about in the previous chapter because it becomes clear from what I have just said that we have another way of talking about crisis. A crisis is our concept of what happens when a person faces a difficulty, either a threat of loss or a loss, in which his existing coping repertoire is insufficient, and he therefore has no immediate way of handling the stress.

During a crisis, even though the person does not have at the start the way of dealing with the problem, he may work out a way of dealing with it before it is over. Some readers may remember those little experiments they used to do years ago in the biology laboratory with a paramecium, where you put a glass plate in front of it, and the paramecium bumps its nose against the glass plate, and then does a lot of trial and error running about to try and find a way around this.

We do the same kind of thing in a crisis. Our existing repertoire is not sufficient, and we try all kinds of things which we did not try before in order to see whether we can handle this situation; and eventually – and this is the peculiar thing about it, I think it has something to do with the homeostatic mechanisms of life – eventually we will find some way. It may be a good way or a bad way, but we will find some way. That is why a crisis does not last longer than about 4 to 6 weeks.

Regression. If there is no solution in reality, or if no solution in fantasy and magic appears to be possible, then the ego is thrown back on a more primitive mechanism still, namely the mechanism of regression. In fact, regression should also include the ways of dealing with a problem by magic and by fantasy. There is a whole range here, from dealing with the problem of the crisis by reality-based means to dealing with it by a wide variety of more and more primitive methods. For instance, the person may deal with it by a kind of childlike magic and wishful thinking, and this may lead to a condition which we recognize as neurosis. Neurosis is a way of dealing with problems by magic, by irrational, symbolic means.

Further regression, if the avenue to neurosis is not open, leads to more primitive disorganization and alienation from the world of reality. The person may deal with difficulties and the tensions associated with them by splitting them off from the rest of his personality; and he splits them off together with a bit of his personality. In other words, in order to avoid facing the tensions that his unified, integrated personality would face if dealing with this unsolved problem, he just smashes up his personality, as it were. This gives him a psychosis. One of the most typical of these is schizophrenia, which was recognized originally by Bleuler as being in essence a splitting, a fragmentation of the personality. If your personality is fragmented you cease to exist from a certain point of view, and cease to feel then the tensions of the unsolved problem. This is a way of escape, and is a quite primitive way. Sometimes there is a complete and absolute disorganization of the personality.

Psychological Work

I want next to come to another concept, that of psychological work. There is an effort involved in psychological operations. In the coping reactions and in the defence reactions psychological effort is involved. When you have to work hard at some problem, you are aware of a certain strain which is not the same as the physical effort of lifting a weight, or something like that, but it makes you tired in a somewhat similar way.

Now, this psychological work is switched on, stimulated, or initiated, by the two main switches in the ego, which I talked

about before. These are the two main ego reactions of anxiety
and depression. Anxiety is one switch, and depression is the other.
Anxiety is the switch that is turned on by threat of loss, and
depression is the switch that is turned on by actual loss.

The psychological work that is switched on by anxiety is called
by some people *worry work* – the work of worrying. The kind of
work that is switched on by depression is known as *grief work*.
The switch is turned on at the beginning of crisis, the *worry work*
or *grief work* takes place during crisis, and then, if the work is
successful, the crisis ends and you get external adaptation. You
mould the external world or adapt it in some way to yourself. At
the same time you get an internal adjustment; your internal
mechanisms have now to take on a novel form to adjust to the
new situation. You had an equilibrium before, then you experienced the hazardous circumstance that constituted the threat, the
switch came into operation, the work was done; during this
period of work there is upset, there is disequilibrium, and you
cannot, at this particular stage, say what is going to happen.
Then, if the work is successful, you get a new equilibrium; and
the new equilibrium has an external aspect – adaptation, and an
internal aspect – adjustment. This adjustment is a relatively lasting condition. In life, whenever you get an equilibrium, it has a
tendency to continue, although I think you have to be aware here
that the concepts of homeostasis do not really apply completely
to human psychology because the human being is in a constant
state of development. My friend, Nathan Ackerman, in his book
on the psychodynamics of family life (1958), talks about *homeo-
dynamics*, not *homeostasis*. After a period of disequilibrium the
equilibrium tends to return not on the same level as it was before,
but always at a step higher in development. Be that as it may,
what we get at the end of crisis is a new equilibrium. The new
equilibrium, if the psychological work has been satisfactory, results in external adaptation and internal adjustment. If the psychological work has not been satisfactory, there is also a new
equilibrium, but this new equilibrium is one of regression. It is a
regressed equilibrium in the direction of either a neurosis, a psychosis, or some form of alienation or disintegration.

43

Anxiety and Worry Work

I want to talk now about anxiety. This is the ego reaction to threat of loss, either of objects or of satisfaction or of integrity. There are two stages of anxiety that can be differentiated quantitatively. First, a small amount of anxiety, which is the initial signal, the sort of little switch that comes on first, is called 'signal anxiety'. This is the reaction that occurs at the initial perception of danger, and is a call to fight or flight. It is a quite primitive biological mechanism. That kind of anxiety has been studied a great deal, and we know that the signal has not only psychological implications, but also physical manifestations, in putting the body rapidly into a state of readiness. The heart-rate changes, the breathing changes, the blood vessels on the skin contract and those in the muscles enlarge, the sugar in the blood goes up, etc., and the body is mobilized to deal with danger. This is signal anxiety.

If the threat is not relieved by the effort to relieve it, and if the danger continues or increases, and if there is no adaptation or adjustment by coping; in other words, if the reality condition continues, and the person does not deal with it – the anxiety increases; and at a certain threshold we say it changes from signal anxiety and becomes what I call 'actual anxiety'.

Anxiety now becomes not a call to action, but a burden. On the other hand, it does have a certain usefulness viewed from a teleological point of view because it forces a new level of ego reaction, namely, the reaction of regression and disintegration. Instead of being a stimulus to fight or to flight or to adjust in an active way, after it passes a certain threshold it becomes a force that squashes the ego into a regressed state of increasing use of fantasy and magic and irrational methods, and then eventually disintegration and alienation, leaving behind, as I said before, the neurosis, psychosomatic illness, or psychosis.

Worry work is the work of internal adjustment stimulated by signal anxiety. It is interesting to turn on the high power of the microscope to look at someone who is doing worry work in order to find out the various factors that may interfere with it. One

44

of the most important factors that interfere with successful worrying is the revival of old memories, of old fantasies of loss, due to previously unsolved conflicts in similar situations. Your previous experience of threat and how you dealt with it rises as a kind of spectre to haunt you when you are now in a state of being stimulated by signal anxiety to do worry work. This is what leads to the effect of childhood experiences in influencing the precipitation in later life of neurosis or psychosis. As we all know, psycho-analysts have paid much attention in past years to the tremendous effect of the way in which one originally solved one's conflicts as a small child on what happens to one in later life in regard to how one deals with threat situations, in determining whether the threat situations precipitate a psychological illness or not. But in addition to the rising of the old spectres, the success of worry work is influenced by a number of factors that are operating in the here-and-now current situation of the threat and of the attempts to grapple with it. Among them one must refer to the current strength of the ego.

This current strength is dependent not only on the person's physical health, but also on something that might be called his constitutional toughness. Some people actually are tougher in dealing with problem situations than others. Strength is dependent not only on these factors, but also on the repertoire of coping responses and on the ability to withstand frustration, which are dependent upon having successfully dealt with past crises.

So in addition to the ego-weakening effects of the revival of old problems during a crisis, you have the ego-strengthening effects of having successfully dealt with crises in the past. This again is common knowledge; how you will deal with a problem now, will depend on whether you have successfully dealt with similar problems in the past. We know that some people, as they go through life, get more and more bowed down, burdened, by one failure after another. If you have had many failures, the chances of failing this time are greater. If you have had many successes, the chances of succeeding this time are greater.

Another factor that will influence the fate of the current problem-solving is the actual environmental danger from a reality

45

point of view; I mean, how dangerous is the situation in actuality? Also, does the stress continue and get worse, or does it start and then finish, or start and get better? If you want to assess what happens in a crisis, it is rather important to know constantly the state of the external reality threat. There is quite a difference, for instance, in the crisis in parents produced by prematurity, where the premature baby is born quite small, but has no congenital abnormalities, and gradually and steadily becomes like an ordinary baby; and in the crisis in parents of a premature baby with a congenital abnormality, which has ups and downs, and some of the downs are quite down. The parents' way of dealing with this situation is determined not only by what is in themselves, but by the ups and down of the external threat situation.

The other factor that is very important in determining the outcome will be the type and degree of environmental support. When a person is dealing with problems, and is in crisis, he is not usually on his own. He has his family around him, he has caretaking agents around him, doctors, nurses, social workers, ministers of religion, etc., who rally round him at that particular moment. This active support and offer of help – as I shall attempt to show in Chapter 5 when I recall some of our observations in Boston on this topic – are a potent factor in determining the outcome.

The outcome of the worry work during the crisis will be a resultant of the interaction of a number of these different forces.

I wish now to go back to something I said before and enlarge on it a little, because probably some readers who have read widely on this subject have been much impressed by the degree of emphasis placed in the past by the psycho-analysts on the effect of unfortunate early childhood experiences on later life situations. I think it is rather important from this point of view to say just a word about how these influences operate. The way they manifest themselves is by weakening the ego currently, because during these past situations there was experience of failure. This experience of failure gets eaten into the person, so that now when he is faced with a difficulty, he has a fantasy of the inevitability of failure. It is this fantasy of the inevitability of failure which weakens him. If you are trying to strengthen someone in the face of difficulty you do not paint a picture that emphasizes that failure is inevitable. If you paint such a picture the person will be weakened. Karl Menninger wrote a paper recently on the importance of hope in psychiatry. Hope is an ego reaction that emphasizes the possibility of success. When you are certain that you are going to fail, you become weaker; and usually you can only stand up and fight if you feel that you have a chance.

Just as a side-issue here, one of the aspects of effective leadership is that the leader, at the moment of danger, increases the ego strength of his followers by painting a picture of the possibility of success. You all remember the magnificent act of leadership of Churchill during the War, after Dunkirk. Although he was painting a picture that appeared to be the picture of 'they're coming over and they're going to kill us all off', the picture that he painted actually was 'We will fight to the last man, and *we will wreak some vengeance on them* – we will fight in the streets, we will fight in the ditches, we will fight in the houses, and we will fight everywhere'. This was the slogan with which he managed to raise the morale of the people of England at that time. In other words, he painted a hopeful picture that, even if we go down, we are going down fighting, and we are going to achieve something even in our going down. We are not just going to lie down and say the situation is hopeless.

The other weakening aspect that is linked to this is the arousal in the present situation of a feeling of guilt, of a feeling of badness, due to old feelings of badness related to those early conflict situations in childhood. There is nothing more weakening than the feeling that one is bad, which means that one deserves punishment; therefore, one deserves defeat. If in childhood there were conflicts which led to solutions such that the child felt constantly guilty thereafter, these conflicts and their solutions usually go underground into the unconscious part of the ego. You forget about them, but when in the future something triggers them off, some crisis situation that resembles one of the earlier crises, the old spectres come out and haunt you and lower your ego strength. This then alters one very important factor in the situation. The

47

point that I want to make here is that *it is only one of the factors.* In addition to the ego weakening due to this, you have the present ego strength, you have the vicissitudes of the reality danger, you have environmental support, and you have something else that I have not mentioned yet, namely, cultural support.

Traditions, and values, and ways of looking at things, and roles, i.e. what you are expected to do, play a very big part in crisis situations and in problem situations. First of all, the very definition of the situation as a problem is partly culturally determined. I was very much impressed once by studying an Italian family, the father of which contracted tuberculosis. I was surprised to discover that, whereas one would expect tuberculosis in the father of a family to produce a major crisis, in this family it did not seem to do so. They did not seem to be very upset. They seemed to say: 'Well, O.K., so he got tuberculosis, he will have to go into a sanatorium, it's the will of God, and we'll pray for him,' but the basis upon which they assessed his functioning as the father of the family was not interfered with by his getting tuberculosis. In many other families, if the breadwinner got tuberculosis, his status as the head of the family would be very much interfered with. The status of this man as the head of the family continued irrespective of his own actions; namely, he was the husband and he was the father of the children, and, therefore, whether he was ill or whether he was well, whether he was a good breadwinner or whether he was not a good breadwinner, whether he was an invalid or whether he was not, he would get all the respect due to him as the head of the household. If they had to go to the hospital to tell him about what was going on and to ask him what to do, that was all right. It was a bit of bother, but his illness produced no alteration in the authority pattern and control mechanisms of the family unit.

Also, the fact that this particular family belonged to a socio-economic group accustomed to disabilities of various kinds – they were used to what some people might call a dependent situation which meant that if they did not earn the money, they would get it through some social agency, and as far as they were concerned you got it either one way or the other – made the father's incapacity less of a burden. You did not live life in their culture in order to do things, in order to earn money, you lived life in order *to be* – in order *to be* happy, in order *to be* a good father, in order *to be* a good child, or in order *to be* a faithful wife. If these were your values in life, tuberculosis was not the tremendously incapacitating hazardous circumstance that it would be to most of us professional people. If we are ill, we are cut off from one of the most important things in our life, which is to do, to succeed, to work, to earn, to rise in status, and so on. So the very definition of the situation is to a considerable extent culturally determined.

Moreover, in certain cultures there are very clear-cut prescriptions of what you should do in particular circumstances. For instance, in that particular family it was clear what you did when you got tuberculosis. You went to church and you prayed, and God would help you if you were good, and they felt that they were good. As far as they were concerned, this way of reacting was laid down by their culture, and this was what they did. They did not feel, as individuals, that they had to work out some individual way of handling this. It was laid down for them.

The cultural definition and the cultural prescriptions and the degree to which this particular threat has been taken into account by the culture are thus likely to be a potent factor in determining what the outcome of worry work will be.

Now, it may be objected, though the culture says that tuberculosis is not a problem, we know that nevertheless it is a problem. After all, the man has to go into the hospital and get cured. He has to take his medicine. What effect is culturally prescribed apathy going to have? I think that you do have to be rather careful sometimes in a case like this, because it is possible for the culture to hamper reality solutions of the problem too. On the other hand, the feeling of ego strength of people in a culture that has already envisaged the problem, and envisaged the solution, their feeling of confidence and ability to do what they have to do, is greater because they do not have to rely entirely on their own individual strength or even on their own family strength. We may think of the culture as a vast external supporting matrix

49

which supports the family, which in turn supports the individual. We shall talk more about this in Chapters 5 and 7.

If worry work is avoided, you get poor adjustment and usually poor adaptation. In other words, faced with a difficulty it is necessary to worry, worrying is purposeful. And if you do not worry, you usually are not stimulated to do the necessary work of adjustment and adaptation. In cases like the one that was mentioned in Chapter 1, where someone in the presence of what should be a crisis just represses all awareness that there is anything wrong, and pretends, either consciously or unconsciously, that things are not wrong, in those circumstances you get disordered behaviour or psychosomatic reactions, in place of dealing with the problem and coping with its psychological consequences. You cannot really play ducks and drakes with reality when it comes down to it. Cultures will usually define as problems those situations which in reality are dangerous, but not always so. Reality is not a purely arbitrary cultural matter. There are certain limits. The culture may decide that it is not important whether you die. If you get tuberculosis and you do not take care of it because your culture prescribes fatalistic inactivity you will die. This may be quite expected in your culture, but people from another culture may feel it to be a sad affair.

Anticipatory Worrying

There is a quite interesting aspect of worry work and of anxiety that it is well to dwell upon. That is the phenomenon of *anticipatory worrying*. When a threat is predicted the person may be able to worry in advance. This anticipatory worrying is quite useful because it relieves the future burden, as long as it is within a controlled range. If it goes overboard, it becomes itself ego-weakening. But if you worry ahead of time at a certain moderate level, you prepare yourself for the situation when it comes. Not only does the person by anticipatory worrying reduce the later burden, but supports, external supports, can be effective in advance by adding to his ego strength, owing to the production of increased confidence in the person in handling the problems when they do appear. 'Forewarned is forearmed.' You usually find, if you consider folk-sayings, that many of the abstruse insights that psychologists produce by much psychological work have an echo in common folk knowledge. The only thing is that folk knowledge is rarely specific, and you will always find a proverb that says the opposite of one that you are quoting, which, I suppose, shows that people realize that flexibility is important in life.

Now, anticipatory support can be specifically engineered by caretaking agents, by a technique which has been known in mental health circles for some time, which we call *anticipatory guidance*. Irving Janis, of Yale, has called it *emotional inoculation*. By this he means building up in advance of the threat a specific resistance to it. The recent work of Janis on emotional inoculation is, I think, of outstanding importance. I would recommend in this context his article in *Psychoanalysis and the Social Sciences* (1958). This describes his researches on patients in a general hospital, and their reactions to surgical operations, and the relationship of their worrying before surgery to their behaviour after surgery. I should like to mention some of the findings of this paper, which I think are quite relevant to the present discussion.

He discovered that if you talk with patients in a surgical ward before their operation, you can classify them almost immediately into three groups. First of all, in Group I, there is an extremely high degree of preoperative fear. These people are constantly worried and agitated, they have marked sleep disturbances, they seek reassurance from authoritative figures but are only momentarily relieved by the reassurance, they attempt to avoid or postpone the operation. In Group II there is moderate anticipatory fear. These are people who are occasionally tense or agitated, they worry about specific features of the operative procedure, or the anaesthesia, but they are relieved when given authoritative assurance. They are able to maintain outward calm most of the time. In Group III, a very interesting group, the people are constantly cheerful and optimistic. They completely deny feeling any concern or worry. There is no observable worry or tension in their behaviour; they sleep well and are able to keep themselves well occupied in reading, socializing, and so on. I suppose that most readers who have worked in surgical wards recognize these three groups.

Janis followed these groups through, and found out what happened after the operations. He found that the persons who were extremely fearful before the operation were more likely than the others to be anxiety-ridden again afterwards. Their excessive fears of body damage were linked with numerous clinical signs of chronic neurotic disturbance. So the excessive worriers before were excessive worriers afterwards. The persons who displayed a moderate degree of preoperative fear were significantly less likely than others to display any apparent form of emotional disturbance during the period of post-operative convalescence. So the moderate worriers before worried least afterwards. And now, the surprising finding – persons who showed a relative absence of preoperative fear were more likely than others to display reactions of anger and intense resentment during post-operative convalescence. The persons that caused the most difficulty for the nurses and surgeons were the group, by and large, who before the operation were most cheerful. The group that had been very worried beforehand remained very worried afterwards. The operation did not very much affect their worries. They continued to worry. They are chronic worriers, and they worry about everything. But of the other two groups, the non-worriers were extremely troublesome afterwards, and the people who had anticipatory worries did best afterwards.

'Many additional observations contribute evidence in support of the following general theoretical proposition: The arousal of anticipatory fear prior to exposure to a stressful life situation is one of the necessary conditions for developing effective inner defenses that enable a person to cope psychologically with the stress stimuli. There is considerable supplementary evidence, which indicates that the nature of the inner defenses that are erected depends upon the degree to which one can overcome the powerful spontaneous tendency to deny the possibility of being personally affected by an impending source of danger. The evidence strongly suggests that if certain (non-denial) types of inner attitudes are formed before the danger materializes the chances of developing traumatic or disorganized symptoms are greatly reduced.

'When we investigate those cases in whom anticipatory fear had been aroused before the operation, we find that they had fantasied or mentally rehearsed various unpleasant occurrences which they had thought would be in store for them. Their anticipated fears seem to have motivated them to seek out and to take account of realistic information about the painful and distressing experiences they would be likely to undergo after waking from anaesthesia and during the period of convalescence. In these persons the conceptions developed prior to the operation often turn out to be essentially correct so that when the unpleasant episodes occur they are not only relatively unsurprised [and surprise in itself is ego weakening], but they feel reassured that events during the recovery phase are proceeding in the expected fashion. [Since the expected fashion leads to recovery, they are reassured further and are strengthened by it.]

'Some individuals [notably those who displayed excessively high anxiety before the operation] appeared to benefit relatively little from having mentally rehearsed the dangers in advance. Most of these cases, as already stated, were persons who chronically suffered from neurotic anxiety, and their post-operative emotional reactions can be regarded as a continuation of their neuroses. Both before and after the operation, they seem to be unable to develop any effective inner defenses to cope with the threat of bodily damage. [We can add, from what we have said already, that the reason for this is that they have deeply imprinted from childhood the inevitability that they are going to be damaged in some kind of symbolic way.]

'Evidently their fears were grounded not so much in the external dangers of surgery as in long-standing unconscious conflicts that were ready to be touched off by any such environmental provocation. But the psychological situation appears to have been quite different among the patients in the moderate anticipatory fear group. These people appeared to be highly responsive to authoritative reassurances from the hospital staff, and seem to have developed a variety of ways and means of reassuring themselves at moments when their fears were strongly aroused. Such patients would frequently report instances of self-reassurance in their post-operative interviews, for example, "I knew that there might be some bad pains, and so when my side started to ache, I told myself that this doesn't mean anything has gone wrong." Such self-reassurances appeared to be rare among the patients who had been relatively free from anticipatory fears before the operation.

[In the third group, the] 'persons remained emotionally calm during the period when they were able to deny the possibility of danger and suffering, but they reacted quite differently as soon as they began to experience the pains and other harassments that accompany the usual recovery from a major surgical operation. They became extremely agitated, and tended to assume that the hospital authorities must be to blame for their suffering. In a few such cases, it seemed quite probable that this way of reacting to external dangers was a manifestation of a characteristic personality tendency' (Janis, 1958, pp. 130–1).

Now, just one or two other excerpts:

'From what has just been said about the dynamics of such behavior one can predict that a number of interrelated adverse affects will ensue if for any reason a person fails to do the work of worrying prior to being exposed to actual danger or loss:

'1. The spontaneous tendency to ward off anticipated fear remains unchecked, and the person therefore remains relatively unmotivated to engage in the realistic fantasying or the mental rehearsing essential for developing two types of effective defenses against fright: (*a*) reality-based cognitions and expectations about opportunities for surviving the impending danger, the subsequent contemplation of which can function as a source of hope and reassurance; and (*b*) reality-based plans for taking protective action in case various contingencies arise, the subsequent execution of which can contribute to reducing feelings of passive helplessness' (Janis, 1958, pp. 141–2).

The important thing to mention here is that when someone feels helpless in the presence of an unpleasant situation, very often what will develop is a feeling of anger and aggressiveness, which then gets turned against outside people who are now, as it were, in loco parentis. The helpless ones blame parental figures for having allowed them to be helpless.

'The person's over-optimistic expectation and fantasies remain uncorrected, and hence the chances are increased that there will be a marked disparity between the amount of victimization expected beforehand and the amount which is actually experienced, increasing the probability of regressive aggrievement reactions' (Janis, 1958, p. 142).

If you watch a little child when he hurts himself, you will find that he often blames his mother, 'You should have protected me and shouldn't allow me to be hurt.' A child feels that whenever anything unpleasant happens it is someone's fault – this is a typical childlike feeling and usually he feels that it is his mother's fault, later on he may internalize it and feel that it is his own fault, because he feels, 'Why did mother allow me to be hurt? Because she doesn't like me. Why doesn't she like me? Because I'm a bad boy. Why am I a bad boy? Because I don't mind her. And I don't like her because she has allowed this bad thing to happen to me. I hate her.' And so it goes on, round and round, and what appears is hatred of mother and hatred of oneself. Because, if one were not bad, mother would protect one.

As Janis says:

'When the person subsequently comes to realize that the danger-control authorities fail to predict or give warning about the suffering that was in store for him, childhood experiences of resentment against the parents (for unfair or unprotective treatment) are especially apt to be reactivated, thus increasing the likelihood that the danger-control authorities will lose their capacity to give reassurances and will be irrationally blamed for objective dangers and deprivations' (Janis, 1958, p. 142).

You can see this is quite a fascinating paper that deserves to be widely read.

The principle that emerges from all of this is that before danger, before a threat situation, people should worry, but they should worry only as much as the reality demands. They should not over-worry, and they should not under-worry. They should worry, in the presence of support, and in an atmosphere of hope. The individual worrying should be in a situation where the external buttressing of the family, of the authority figures, and of the caretaking agents of society, gives him the strong possibility of a hopeful outcome.

This then leads us to be able to say something about the techniques of anticipatory guidance. In giving anticipatory guidance to people before an event which you predict is going to be dangerous, the important point is to stress the real detail of what they will perceive. You do not have to go into all the painful possibilities of what they are not likely to perceive. The thing to do is to talk about the things that you know they are likely to hear, and feel, and smell afterwards. It should not be just a nice story. I am sickened sometimes by reading some of the stuff put out by people who try anticipatory guidance and sugar it all up and make it completely useless. There is one book that was produced to prepare children to go into hospital. If you read this book you would think that going to hospital was the most wonderful thing in the world. People there play with you and there are nice toys and you get ice-cream after the operation, and so on; and by the time you finish the book you really feel that going into hospital is a wonderful thing. The only thing is that when you get into the hospital it is not going to be like that.

And so the net effect of this book, supposing anyone ever read it and took it to heart, and I very much hope they did not, would be to increase the feeling of victimization afterwards because the child would now feel that he had been told a lie, which he had. The important thing is to state realities, and the painful realities as they will be felt, but at the same time to show a way of handling them, and a picture of the support and the help and the reassurance that will come along the way, and of the hope of successful outcome within the range of predictive reality.

Let us take one of the very difficult things like trying to help someone who is going to die. Of course it is hard to generalize about this topic, and each case must be judged on its merits with due regard to the personalities of the people involved, but there are certain principles which can guide action. It is usually no use giving a hopeful outcome to someone who has got a short time to live – neither to him, nor to the people around him. On the other hand, there are certain limits to the catastrophe that is impending. It is not the end of the world, it is going to be the end of this person, but it is not going to be the end of his relations or his family, of his accomplishments in life, and so on. What one tries to do in this is to paint reality undistorted by dreams and fantasies; and, after all, the remarkable thing is that it is not reality that makes cowards of people, it is dreams. It is dreams that make cowards of us all – nightmares, of course, not nice dreams. If one can remove the nightmare quality, and at the same time help them face reality, people really have a tremendous resilience and a tremendous amount of strength. It also helps to deal with them as people of their age, and not as children.

I should like to add one or two things about the topic of anxiety. I think that one should differentiate between fear and anxiety. Fear is a reaction to present danger. Anxiety is a reaction to the idea of danger. It is an abstract concept. And since it is abstract it is more easily influenceable by other abstractions such as fantasies.

I would also make mention of the phenomenon of apathy. Apathy may be due to an unawareness of danger, and it is a source of difficulty because it prevents anticipatory worrying. But

57

apathy may also be a defence by denial of extreme anxiety with which the person refuses to or cannot cope. In a group of apathetic people, there are therefore two sub-categories. The first comprises those who just do not realize there is going to be a danger, and the second consists of those who understand only too well and just cannot cope with it. If you try to deal with the apathetic group by stimulating all of them to get an increased awareness of danger, you will get a paradoxical reaction in one sub-category. In the group that are apathetic because they do not realize there is a danger, stimulation increases effectiveness, because they will do some anticipatory worrying. In the group who are apathetic as a defence by denial of the difficulties of the situation, the more you stimulate them by painting a picture of the dangers, the more apathetic they will get. This reminds me of Middlemore's studies on babies at the breast. Middlemore, in *The Nursing Couple,* describes how she sat on the beds of mothers nursing their newborn infants and watched the behaviour of the mother and of the baby at the breast. She classified babies into satisfied sucklings and unsatisfied sucklings; and among the unsatisfied sucklings there was a group of apathetic, sleepy babies, as everyone who has worked in a newborn nursery knows. People tried to stimulate them by flicking their toes, or pinching them, or slapping their bottoms to wake them up, and some of the babies would wake up. If you flicked their toes they would start sucking. But with some of the babies, the more you flicked their toes the deeper they went to sleep. These were the ones who were somnolent and withdrawn as a reaction to extreme sensitivity. They could not bear stimulation and so they retired into themselves. The more you stimulated them the more they retired.

This reminds me of certain schizophrenics who are stuporose. If you try to wake them from their stupor, the more you try and wake them up, the deeper they go into stupor; because the stupor is an active defence against the world by turning into the self.

Depression and Grief Work

Now, I have space for only a brief discussion of depression. This is the second main ego reaction. It is the reaction to loss of an object, or loss of integrity. It is manifested by pain, by emptiness, and by a feeling of helplessness. The loss of the object is what occurs in bereavement situations, when someone dies, or in a disappointment. You can be depressed as a result, for instance, of some loved one suddenly behaving in a quite unexpected way, which is disappointing. The disappointment of lovers is a typical situation in which depression and reactions like bereavement occur. Loss of integrity is also a cause. One often finds depression after, for instance, loss of a limb, or very frequently, after the loss of the uterus, after hysterectomy. Hysterectomy is a typical situation of loss of an essential part of one's being, and practically everyone who has a hysterectomy passes through a period of depression.

Like anxiety, there are two levels. There is first of all what I call 'signal depression'. It stimulates the ego to do grief work, and to adjust and adapt to the loss. And secondly there is 'actual depression'. If the grief work is not satisfactory and the loss continues, then the deepening depression becomes an ego burden and leads to ego-weakening, to regression, to disintegration, to alienation. These are the cases that lead on to a depressive psychosis.

As with worry work, grief work is interfered with by previously unsolved problems, especially those relating to conflict of love and hate in relation to a love-object. The solution of these conflicts is a very essential part of the development of one's feelings of relationship with other people. An infant has to cope with a mixture of internal instinctual drives, some of them towards love, and some of them towards hate and destruction. This primitive internal conflict of love and hate appears in the earliest relationship of the infant to his mother, and the way in which this conflict is dealt with will determine how his personality develops and how he is able to love others. In loving others, there is never pure love, it is always mixed with some hate. The question is which is preponderant. How one loves others will also have an echo in how one loves oneself. So the person who is unable to love others is unable also to love himself, and he hates himself as well as hating others. It is the hate of oneself which weakens one, as I said earlier, because it produces a feeling of badness, of inevitability of punishment and destruction and doom.

There can be anticipatory grieving in the same way as anticipatory worrying, and to some extent it works in a positive way by lightening the subsequent load. But sometimes it causes trouble, and that is if the loss does not occur. You have already gone some distance towards adjusting that person out of your life. This is not infrequent in the case of a returning soldier where the wife and the rest of the family have anticipated that he is going to get killed, and they have dealt with this by closing their lives off from him. When he comes back, he is a stranger. There is a complicated process necessary then of bringing the object back into one's life after it has been extruded. Not only does this happen to soldiers who go to the war, but it also happens to a lesser extent to people who go off to prolonged hospitalizations, either to a mental hospital or to a TB hospital or to some other hospital for chronic illnesses. When they go they are lost, and the family mourns, and does its grief work, but then when they come back they have to be reborn again, as it were, in this family.

Healthy grieving has been very well described by Eric Lindemann, and I give a reasonably full account of this in Chapter 8, so I feel less guilty that I am rushing through this discussion so quickly here. Healthy grieving lasts from about four to six weeks, and it has certain characteristic signs and symptoms, insomnia, loss of interest in the surroundings, loss of appetite, constipation, a painful feeling of emptiness, weeping, sighing respirations, and preoccupation with the image of the lost one. Grief work consists essentially in reviewing one's life with the person who is dead, or who is lost; and piecemeal, bit by bit, actively renouncing the gratifications of the past association. When you mourned, and I suppose most people have had the experience of mourning, you remember you constantly thought over how you went here or there with mother or father, and how nice it was, and then you realized little by little each time that no longer would you be able to go with mother or father, or sister or brother, or whoever it was, and do these things in that way. From now on, you have to do them alone or with someone else. There is a beautiful song by

Mahler in his *Kindertotenlieder*. This is a series of poems about two children who died. In one of the poems, which is set to beautiful music, the poet describes how the father sees the mother coming in through the door, and his eye goes down to the level where he would see the head of his daughter as she comes in holding her mother's hand; and he looks at the door, and he sees his wife coming in, and where the child's head should be, there is nothing. He sits and he weeps as he remembers this, and he imagines the mother coming in with the little girl, and now he sees her coming in, and there is no little girl. And he cries, 'From now on, when mother comes through the door, you will not be there.' This is painful, it is a reviewing of the situation, and it is an active act of resignation. He becomes resigned to the inevitable that never more will the little girl come through the door in that way.

The essence of grief work consists of psychologically burying the dead. In unhealthy grieving, you find people who show a false happiness, or a simple denial. They just deny and say, 'Well, so what, so-and-so died', or they even say, 'He didn't die', and they do not believe he did. There is a very characteristic inability to picture the lost one. They cannot do what Mahler did, look at the mother and imagine the figure of the little girl.

This leads almost inevitably to disorder. The disorder that follows unhealthy grieving is usually a psychosomatic illness, such as ulcerative colitis. Many cases of ulcerative colitis are precipitated by loss and by unhealthy grieving, or by inability to grieve about loss. Inadequate grieving may lead to character change, in which the person who is alive takes on the characteristics, or some of the characteristics, of the dead one; as though he has taken him into himself, and now he says, 'My father didn't die, he continues to live because he lives through me.' And you will find sometimes that wives of famous men, when their husbands have died, suddenly change their profession. They take on the profession of the dead man, and they move around as though they were the famous person. The widow is quite out of keeping with reality, but she feels that the husband continues to live as though he lives through her. In the same way that in unhealthy worrying there was free-floating aggression, in unhealthy grieving, too, there is a good deal of hostility and aggression which are directed at the people around, especially at the people who might be thought to be responsible for something which caused the death of the person. The aggression is either directed against them or directed against oneself. 'I caused my brother's death; I should have done this, or that, or the other.'

Caretaking agents can help people to grieve adequately, they can support them. No one likes to be in pain, and in order to put up with pain, you need support, or at least it helps to be supported. People can be urged to do the grief work. They can be educated on how they should review their life with the lost one. They can be encouraged and supported in burying the dead.

Interestingly enough, in most religions an important aspect of the religious tradition consists in helping people to do grief work in this kind of way. And an important aspect of religion is also to help people to do worry work.

My final point is this. It is not necessary to analyse the reasons for the difficulty in doing grief work. If you find people who are not grieving adequately, you do not have to analyse their childhood experiences and fantasies to find what it is that went on years ago which now may be contributing to the fact that they are not grieving adequately. Those factors are linked with deep unsolved past conflicts, usually of mixed relationships of love and hate with a previous loved one, or with this particular loved one. You do not have to analyse all that. All you have to do is to support the people and help them in order to make sure that they do in fact do the psychological work of grieving and burying their dead at the present time.

In concluding this presentation I would like to say that I am sorry I have burdened you with so much theory in the last two chapters, but I feel that we can now turn to more practical matters during the remainder of the book, with the knowledge that we share a certain conceptual framework which we can use as a focal point for our discussion of the problems of our daily work with children and their families. I know I have had to cover a great deal of ground, perhaps a little too rapidly for easy comprehension, but I hope some of you will find an opportunity to learn more about these matters through reading the works to which I have made reference.

REFERENCES

ACKERMAN, NATHAN (1958). *The Psychodynamics of Family Life.* New York: Basic Books.

CAPLAN, GERALD (1959). *Concepts of Mental Health and Consultation.* Washington, D.C.: Children's Bureau Publication No. 373.

FREUD, ANNA (1937). *The Ego and the Mechanisms of Defence.* London: Hogarth; New York: International Universities Press.

JANIS, IRVING L. (1958). 'Emotional Inoculation: Theory and Research on Effects of Preparatory Communications.' In *Psychoanalysis and the Social Sciences.* New York: International Universities Press.

MIDDLEMORE, M. P. (1941). *The Nursing Couple.* London: Hamish Hamilton.

CHAPTER 3

The Psychology of Pregnancy, and the Origins of Mother-Child Relationships

PREGNANCY AND CRISIS

I SHALL start off by relating what I am going to say here to the discussions of the last two chapters; and the first word that comes to mind is the word *crisis*. What is the relation of our theory of crisis to pregnancy?

I suppose that from a certain point of view you could think of the whole period of pregnancy as a period of crisis. It has certain aspects that are similar to the definitions of crisis that I have developed during the past two chapters. It is a period of altered behaviour; it is a period of disequilibrium compared with the normal state of the family; it is a period of emotional upset in the woman, and often in her husband and her other children. It is a period when there are problems, many of which cannot be adequately handled by the use of the customary problem-solving mechanisms. Yet it does not quite fit into our concept of crisis, because it is really rather too long. Forty weeks is too long to conceive of as a crisis; and moreover, you get the feeling of an equilibrium during the period itself. The period has, as it were, a stable life of its own.

Nevertheless, if you look at the period of pregnancy, one thing strikes you, and that is that the susceptibility to intercurrent crises seems to be greater than usual. And as we look at this period it reminds us of certain other manifestations in the life process, namely the period of adolescence and the period of the climacterium. Both of these periods have a pattern of their own, different from the behavioural pattern before and after, and both of them seem to be tumultuous periods, periods of emotional reverberations, you might say. In both these periods people get upset in characteristic ways for relatively short periods. So probably the best way to think of the period of pregnancy is as a period of increased susceptibility to crisis. In which case we have to ask ourselves how we explain this in the light of what we have been saying above.

We might suppose that if we find a period of increased susceptibility to crisis we would expect, on the one hand, the emergence of an increased number of hazardous circumstances, an increased number of important problems which represent a threat or a loss, or an obstacle to gratification of life's goals; and, on the other hand, we might expect either that there will be a weakening of the essential ego structure, so that the person cannot make use of his usual repertoire of problem-solving methods, or that his supports in his family, in his social environment, and in his culture, might be weakened; and, therefore, he is less able than usual to deal with these problems.

These are, I suppose, some of the possibilities First of all, this is certainly a period when problems of an important nature appear to be present in increased degree. One of the most important of these problems is that the woman is preparing for a completely new role. If this is her first baby, she is moving from being a wife to becoming a mother. If it is her second baby, she is changing from being a mother of one child to becoming a mother of two. I suppose that one would expect the problems to be greater for the woman who is having her first baby, because the change from being a wife to becoming a mother is usually greater than the change from being a mother of one child to becoming a mother of two. But in certain circumstances, becoming the mother of two children may be quite a good deal more complicated a situation than being the mother of one.

We must realize that, in preparing for this new role, it is likely that there will be the revival of old ideas and fantasies of what this role may entail. And if we are talking about the woman who is having her first baby, then she has probably carried within her from the days of her girlhood certain ideas and hopes and expectations of what it will mean to become a mother. And these hopes and expectations will not be entirely uncomplicated. Surely she will have hopes of becoming a good mother; but if, for instance, in her past life, the model of mother, namely her own mother, was someone with whom she had a conflictual relationship, then, when she thinks of becoming a mother herself, the complications of that early relationship are likely to come to the surface. They are likely to modify her feelings about what will happen when she becomes a mother and, as it were, takes her mother's place. Will she be a better mother than her own mother was or will she be worse?

In addition to that, there are the problems associated with the fact that pregnancy is a very prominent, and increasingly prominent, manifestation that this girl has had sexual intercourse. If the girl has had complications in her feelings about herself as a sexual person, then these are likely to be stimulated during the period of pregnancy. She walks around, as it were, saying to the world, 'I am a person who has had sexual intercourse.' This may arouse in her complicated feelings of anxiety, shame, and guilt.

It is therefore likely that for some women there is an increased susceptibility to crisis, because of the increase of certain problems. These problems are not entirely of a psychological nature; there are economic and social problems involved too, of which we should not lose sight. In our culture, especially in urban situations and especially with a young married couple, the advent of a baby is a complicated issue from an economic and social point of view. Nowadays, when it seems to be the custom for the wife as well as the husband to work, the idea that she has to interrupt her working-life is a matter of no small consequence. In our practice in Boston we dealt with quite a large number of students, where the wife was working to put her husband through college. The whole family future depended upon his being able to continue through school and graduate to become a professional person; and this in turn depended upon the income the wife was producing. Pregnancy in those circumstances became a rather difficult problem, if the couple consciously had decided that they were going to postpone having a baby, and then there was either some real mistake or some 'mistake' on purpose by one or the other of them. This was sure to arouse feelings of guilt, and often represented a major interference with their carefully worked-out plans.

In addition, there are the difficulties of housing. A couple can often get accommodation if they have no children. If they have children it is harder to do so, and, of course, there is the increased expense at a time when the earning capacity of the family goes down. So, obviously, a number of such problems are apt to crop up, and these may colour the whole situation in a pregnancy. Unless we take these into account, we cannot really understand what is going on. It is not just the simple biological situation of a woman having a baby.

Now, let us look at the other side of the equation – the ego strength, the capacity to use the repertoire of problem-solving methods in order to deal with these problems. This is altered in a rather complex way during pregnancy, mainly due to the metabolic changes of the period. A physician said to me recently that he likes my term 'somatopsychic'. When I use this term I am talking about something that is quite different from 'psychosomatic'. The familiar terms 'psychosomatic' refers to secondary bodily effects of primary psychological processes. When I talk about 'somatopsychic' reactions, I am talking about secondary psychological manifestations of processes that are primarily bodily. Both these words are rather silly, because they imply a dualism; they imply that there are bodily processes and psychological processes; that these are quite separate; and that one set of processes affects the other set of processes. Whereas most of us nowadays look upon the manifestations of behaviour as the manifestations of a unitary organism. Every manifestation can be conceived of from the point of view both of the organic processes and of the psychological processes. It depends which instrument you are using to inspect the behaviour and record the phenomena. If you are using psychological instruments, then you bring into focus the psychological manifestations. If you are using an organic instrument, then you uncover somatic manifestations.

Whatever is going on can always be looked at from one or other point of view. No doubt the only reason for using these terms is that the manifestations that seem to be exciting, at least to the observer, can alter from situation to situation. That is to say, at certain times the organic changes seem to be exciting; at other times, the psychological changes seem to be exciting. This is really a fallacy, because I personally am usually excited by the psychological manifestations, and my colleagues who specialize more in the physical aspects of health and illness are more excited by the organic changes.

Nevertheless, from the point of view of exposition, it may be useful to think in these terms, although we should be aware of our artificial dualistic approach. This is just a way of talking in order to describe the processes and to tease out the equation.

One of the characteristics of pregnancy, which it shares with the climacterium and to some extent with adolescence, is the tumultuous change that takes place in the body metabolism. This can be expressed in its simplest form by the hormonal changes. There are all kinds of complex hormonal changes which take place from conception through to after delivery. I would like to emphasize that the changes continue till *after* delivery.

I am no expert on the metabolic changes that take place, but from where I sit, it seems as though there is a continuous change during the forty weeks of pregnancy and afterwards. We have a certain amount of evidence to show that, when hormonal changes occur, they are accompanied by complicated psychological changes.

I was talking about the psychological aspects of pregnancy in the Medical School at New Orleans a few months ago; and in their Department of Psychiatry they have been doing some quite interesting work on the aetiology of schizophrenia. They have isolated certain biochemical products from the blood and urine of schizophrenic patients which do not occur in normal people, and which when injected into normal volunteers produce schizophrenia-like psychotic symptoms. They are very interested, in New Orleans, in the metabolic aetiological factors of psychosis. I had been talking to the workers in this department during the previous couple of days about preventive psychiatry, and they seemed quite interested; but as I began talking about the psychological aspects of pregnancy, I noticed that the whole audience were sitting on the edge of their chairs. I wondered what was going on because they did not look like people who had any special interest in the problems of pregnancy. And then it occurred to me as I went on, and as the discussion opened, that in my description of what takes place during pregnancy, and of the relation of the normal metabolic changes in pregnancy to psychological changes, these psychiatrists were recognizing certain manifestations with which they were familiar in the pathological field, in regard to metabolic changes that are either the cause or the accompaniment of some of the changes in schizophrenia. This was especially so when I talked about a peculiar change that we have found in pregnancy where the irrational fantasy forces of the id, as it were, erupt into the ego area. I shall talk about this shortly. This is exactly, from a certain point of view, what occurs in schizophrenia; and this is what they have found when they inject these schizophrenia substances into normal volunteers. The rational ways of thinking of the latter are invaded by irrational processes and irrational ways of looking at reality. Later on, as we continued with the discussion, someone mentioned that one of the peculiar chemical products found in the urine of schizophrenia patients had also been isolated in the urine of pregnant women.

Now, this is beginning to take me into a subject that I do not know much about, so I will keep quiet about it, except just to mention that there is the possibility that in normal pregnancy there are certain metabolic changes which resemble some of the pathological changes that are found in psychotics. This then links up with the independent finding that if you take a close look at the pregnant woman, a much closer look than anyone has taken in the past, you find that there are certain aspects of her psychological functioning that resemble the psychological functioning of certain psychotic patients. Of course, there are very important differences, which I shall come to later.

So a prediction based upon the theories presented in the last two chapters, that one would find in a period of increased susceptibility to crisis (*a*) more problems and (*b*) an altered capacity to deal with problems, seems to be borne out by our examination of what actually does take place in pregnancy.

What about the third point that I made, namely, the weakening of external supports to the ego in regard to dealing with these problems? Here we are on more uncertain ground, but I think that we do have something to say. The upsets in the pregnant woman, as a result of all that she is going through, are apt to produce upsets in the equilibrium of all members of her family, particularly her husband. The upsets produced in him are upsets in his relationship with his wife, so that very often he is less able to support her during this period than during their normal relationship when she is not pregnant.

In most cultures, pregnancy and birth are periods to which the culture pays particular attention. There are all kinds of traditions and customs and ways of people rallying around, and prescriptions of things to do and things not to do, some of which sound to us like superstitions. But superstitions are part of a culture. If you examine it closely, you will discover that the superstition has some very special meaning. I do not propose to go into this in detail, but what I want to emphasize is that in well-established cultures, the pregnant woman is enveloped in a series of prescriptions of what she should do, what she should not do, what other people should do to her, what they should not do to her, and so on, which is more marked than in her ordinary life.

A special aspect of the United States is that, at the present time and for some time past, the country has been a melting-pot of cultures. There are other parts of the world at the present time which are also cultural melting-pots where there is rapid culture change, especially the pioneer countries, and the rapidly developing countries. One would expect that in these circumstances the external supports of the culture would be weakened. Therefore, I would expect that the pregnant woman would be more susceptible to crises in such a culture in transition than she would be if she were enmeshed and enveloped in a stable culture where everyone knew exactly what to do and did it without too much question. So I would say that probably in the United

States and in a number of other countries in the world at the present time, owing to the tremendous increase in the speed of communication, and to a general breaking down of the old cultural boundaries that separated one culture from another, pregnancy is becoming a more upsetting period than perhaps it used to be. It would be very interesting to do some research to confirm this.

If, then, pregnancy is a period of increased susceptibility to crisis because of all these reasons, what significance does this have for us in the light of what I have been saying above? There are two aspects of crisis that we must particularly take into account.

(1) In a crisis, old problems are brought to the surface and new problems are faced, and there is the possibility at this time of novel solutions which may be in a healthy direction, or in an unhealthy direction.

(2) A person in crisis, because of the disequilibrium, because the situation is in a state of flux, is more susceptible to influence than when he is not in crisis.

Therefore, we can say that the crises of pregnancy present us with a very good opportunity to affect, by minimal intervention, the future mental health of the woman. And since we are dealing here with a series of crises which are strung on the strand of the development of the relationship of this woman to her future child, this gives us an unequalled opportunity to influence the way that she will develop in her relationship as a future mother to this child. Moreover, since the crises involve in an intimate way not only the woman but all the rest of the family, this gives us an opportunity to intervene by the use of minimal effort, in order to improve the total family relationships of this little group of people. It is from these points of view that I am interested in the psychology of pregnancy.

EMOTIONAL CHANGES IN PREGNANCY

Now I shall very briefly run through some of the factual information that we have about the changes in normal pregnancy. I am going to be brief because I realize that it is familiar to most readers. First of all, let me say just one other word in introduction. In order to talk about the emotional changes in pregnancy we have to specify what stage of pregnancy we are discussing, because there is a dynamic unfolding in the psychological area in the same way as in the physical area during pregnancy. There are certain changes which we recognize as occurring in the first trimester, in the second trimester, and in the third trimester. And I feel that it is very important for me again to emphasize that the study of the psychology of pregnancy should not end at delivery. There should be a follow-through, because this is a continuous process going through to the life of the woman afterwards, and certainly going through to the first three or four weeks after delivery. Delivery is one element of the unfolding process.

Mood Swings

Among the characteristic changes which take place during pregnancy, as you all know, are peculiar and apparently unexplainable changes in dominant mood, and mood swings. These occur usually fairly early in pregnancy, and have a variable course throughout the whole period including the post-partum period. The woman may become elated or depressed. She is not depressed because she did not want to become pregnant; and she is not elated because she did want to become pregnant. Women who wanted to become pregnant may be depressed, and women who did not want to become pregnant find themselves elated. These mood changes seem to be very closely connected with complicated swings and alterations of the metabolic process. Associated with these is an increased sensitivity in most areas of the woman's functioning. This is shown emotionally. She has very quickly changing feelings and shows increased irritability; she gets angry more frequently, and she cries more easily. She shows increased sensitivity – a woman who was usually a stable person will become very sensitive to slights. She may laugh more easily than before. She is more sensitive in all areas, not just in these predominantly psychological areas, but also in taste, and smell, and hearing. Pregnant women tend to get disgusted very easily at unpleasant smells or tastes. A peculiarity of these changes is that they occur in waves. The woman may be irritable one day, and not the next; sensitive one day, and not the next; sensitive one week, and not the next. It is as if a cloud is lifting up and down, which is very characteristic of organically induced psychological changes, as we know from general psychiatry. In, for example, disorders of the cortex, in senility, in senile dementia, or pre-senile dementia, or in a toxic process, you see this cloud-like rising and lowering from minute to minute, or from hour to hour, or from week to week. I have had this same feeling in mountain regions in regard to my feeling of sleepiness. One minute you are feeling sleepy, and the next you are feeling alert again; and then half an hour later you are feeling sleepy again. This is, I think, the resultant of the altitude and the change of climatic conditions. I do not think it is due to direct environmental stimulation, because if you are bored, and if you are sleepy because of fatigue, then the fatigue gets progressively deeper and deeper. You do not go up and down in this way.

Appetite

Another, and well-recognized, peculiarity of pregnancy is change of appetite. People talk about it mainly from the point of appetites for food, the food cravings that go up and down in strange ways. I am not thinking at present of the increased appetite characteristic of many pregnant women, which I shall discuss in a moment, but of sudden changes in appetite. There is one area which is rather important for us, from the point of view of preventive psychiatry, and that is the change in sexual appetite. One of the characteristics of pregnancy is the change which may take place in this area, and which varies from woman to woman and from time to time during pregnancy. A woman who may have had a relatively low sexual appetite may now have a greater sexual appetite, and a woman who had a high sexual appetite may lose it. Not only is there a change in appetite, there is a change in the whole functioning of sex, such as a change in sexual performance, so that the woman who previously had a gratifying sex life may now find herself 'frigid'. You also find

74

women who have orgasms for the first time during pregnancy, or some who have orgasms only during pregnancy.

This is sometimes associated with the increased euphoria of pregnancy, so that you sometimes find women who become 'pregnancy addicts'. I know a couple of them. They feel better during pregnancy than at any other time, and they look better too. There is one young lady that we know in Boston, who somewhat shamefacedly came back to our Family Health Clinic time after time. When she was not pregnant, she appeared quite a decent-looking woman. But during pregnancy, she was absolutely beautiful; she looked and felt radiant; and everything about her rose to a high ecstatic peak, including her sexual performance. I hope that one day, with the help of our colleagues who are specialists in the metabolism of pregnancy, we shall be able to discover exactly what biochemical process leads to these changes which occur in some women and not in others, and at certain times and not at others. This would be a fascinating and important contribution to the whole theory of the aetiology of mental illness, and of mental health.

Introversion and Passivity

The other characteristic and very well-recognized aspect of pregnancy is the introversion and passivity of the pregnant woman. This is very common; it begins about the end of the first trimester, and gradually increases in intensity to reach a peak about the seventh or eighth month. Women who have been outgoing, active people now wish to sit and receive, instead of giving. They turn in on themselves. The sentimental picture of the pregnant woman sitting in passive contemplation, and knitting away at little baby clothes; or the less sentimental picture of the pregnant woman who wants to lie in bed and have her husband bring her breakfast to her; these are manifestations of this introversion and passivity. Some women like it; they feel that this makes them more relaxed, they do not have to go rushing about all the time. Some women resent it intensely. They say, 'I don't like this, I feel like a cow; I feel lazy; I can't put up with this.' This latter group of women represents a difficulty from the point of view of

75

management, because it would appear that the introversion and passivity are almost certainly caused by the metabolic changes in pregnancy and are a very necessary psychological stage in preparation for adequate motherhood. Nature, as it were, produces a situation where the woman, in preparing to be a giving person to her future infant, passes first of all through a preparatory stage of being a receiving person. There is a certain amount of evidence that those women who do not get what they ask for during pregnancy afterwards have difficulty in giving, when the infant asks from them.

The pregnant woman is especially susceptible to any disorder in her family which results in her not getting what she demands during pregnancy. And she visits this, unconsciously, upon the baby afterwards. If she has been deprived during pregnancy, she cannot be a giving person afterwards, and she deprives her infant.

The group of women who rebel against the passivity of pregnancy also seem to have trouble afterwards. This is not so for all of them, but there is more trouble in that group than in the group that accepts the 'cow-like condition', and does not even call it cow-like. The former women are in a conflict, they are fighting with themselves; and as you listen to them talking, they talk about it as a fight; they feel this impulse pressing down upon them to make them lazy and passive, and they just cannot bear it. They have to fight. Those are the women, by and large, who have certain personality characteristics involving conflicts over their femininity. The feminine role in our culture was traditionally the sort of lady-like role of waiting for a man to open a door for her. It does not quite work out that way nowadays, but this is the general concept of the role of woman; and there are certain girls who already in childhood are rebelling against it. They demand to open the door for themselves. Our culture now rewards activity on the part of women. Women are no longer supposed to be gentle little ladies who swoon and have vapours, and so on. They are sometimes supposed to go out and earn the money so that their husbands can study. But this means that women who have conflicts over their femininity are encouraged to seek a rebellious solution of the problem by activity, by being equal to men, by going out and doing, and by achieving. When they become pregnant and have to give up this role, they regard this as something alien to their whole personality situation. And so they fight against it, and if they cannot be persuaded by us to relax and let nature take its course, the fight continues afterwards, and they have difficulty later on in playing the appropriate maternal role in regard to the infant. Now this is a little peculiar, because after all, the role in relation to the infant is an active, giving role. And yet as we look a little closer at what goes on between a mother and her infant, for instance in the breast-feeding situation, we find that in order for there to be a really relaxed relationship, the mother must be able to play two roles. On the one hand she is giving to the infant and, on the other hand, she is identifying with the infant at her breast. If you watch a really satisfactory mother-child relationship in a young mother feeding her infant, you will notice the mother almost does not have to look at the infant to know what the infant is feeling. She feels it herself; and she is both the giver of the milk and, as it were, the receiver of the milk. The peculiar harmony of that picture is produced by the fact that this is really a circular process. In order to be able to play those two roles, she has to have the ability to give while being in a receptive mood. And she is, as it were, rehearsing this all the way through pregnancy. This is just my theory, but it is certainly a fact that women who have difficulty accepting the introversion of pregnancy have difficulties afterwards in the earliest relationships with their babies.

Change in Ego-Id Equilibrium

Now we come to a phenomenon which, apart from the writings of our little group in Boston, has not received much attention so far in the literature. I predict, however, that it will receive increased attention over the next few years. I refer to what I have called the change in equilibrium between the ego and the id. We happened on it almost by accident when we asked a psychologist to do some personality tests on a number of normal pregnant women; and we were rather surprised when he turned in reports saying that they were all very seriously emotionally disturbed. He suspected schizophrenia. But they did not quite fit the schizophrenia picture, because there was no defect in reality-testing, that is to say, the women knew what was fact and what was fancy, but they had the kind of fancies that usually only schizophrenics have. We were rather upset about this, and so we asked another psychologist to test some other women, and he came up with a similar result. A third psychologist also produced the same result. Then we realized that what we were dealing with was a normal manifestation, which had apparently escaped notice because no one had taken the trouble to use these tests on a group of normal pregnant women before. This fitted in with something else we had noticed. Beginning at the end of the first trimester, and increasing all the way through pregnancy, continuing for about two or three weeks post-partum, and then disappearing, pregnant women, if they feel that you will listen sympathetically to them, will voice all kinds of peculiar fantasies that have a dream-like quality and are not at all the kind of talk that characterizes their normal non-pregnant condition.

Moreover, we find, especially near the middle and towards the end of pregnancy, a very interesting revival of early childhood memories of old conflicts. Conflicts such as a woman may have had with her mother when she was a little girl, or with her sisters or brothers, or her father, which had been repressed and forgotten, emerge into consciousness, and the woman becomes preoccupied with them. In addition, interestingly enough, usually about the end of the second trimester, old conflicts about her sex life, and particularly about masturbation, that she had during adolescence and in earlier life begin to emerge. She will talk about these things which she had forgotten before, and she will dream about them. The interesting thing is how openly she talks about material which a psycho-analyst might say would usually take a couple of years of analysis to bring to the surface. Moreover, she talks with relatively little·anxiety about material which you would expect her to be very anxious about. Not only does she talk to you in this way, but you can talk very openly to her. Visitors who have sat in while I have been interviewing pregnant women,

78

especially towards the middle and end of pregnancy, have often been quite amazed and shocked at the way in which I talk to them so openly about problems of masturbation, problems of relationships with their mothers, and so on. I have found that free discussion of this kind of material with a pregnant woman is perfectly in order.

It reminds one somewhat of the way one can talk to a schizophrenic. Schizophrenics have a remarkable aptitude for understanding symbolism. They can talk to you quite directly about irrational material, and they can make interpretations of a symbolic nature that you would expect usually only in an experienced psycho-analyst or analysand. The reason for this is that, in the ordinary personality, there are repressing forces which keep down the irrational fantasy material in the id and in the unconscious parts of the ego, but in the schizophrenic there is a disintegration of personality, and the repressing forces are weakened, so that the irrational material comes up to the surface of consciousness. In the presenting personality of a schizophrenic you are dealing with his ego all mixed up with his id. In the ordinary person, in order to release these forces of the unconscious, you have to do a lot of hard work as a psycho-analyst, to chip away at the repressing forces, and little by little to allow the irrational material to come up to the surface. In pregnancy it seems to happen spontaneously. The interesting question is why people did not recognize this phenomenon before.

I think that pregnant women, as a group, recognize that these ideas which are coming into their minds are a bit crazy. They recognize that other people would think they were very strange, and they usually do not tell people about them. They tell each other about them. One of the phenomena of pregnancy of which I am sure you are all aware is the way in which pregnant women cluster together. If you listen to what they are saying, and if they go on talking while you are there, it raises the hair on your head to hear the monstrous stories that they tell each other. This has long been recognized in a negative way by people who run classes for pregnant women. I never used to be able to understand why sophisticated people running classes for expectant mothers never gave the expectant mothers a chance to talk, or only allowed them to talk about very clearly defined subjects. If you look at the Red Cross guide on mothers' classes you will find that there is no possibility for the expectant mother to talk, because the nurse who is running the course has so much material to cover in each session, most of it so very highly structured that all the expectant mothers can do is to ask direct questions and get factual answers. Usually what happens in classes which I have observed is that when some woman begins to talk about something that has a slightly irrational flavour, the person who is running the group puts the damper on and says, 'Well, that's just a lot of superstition, you don't have to bother about that, etc., etc.,' and gives some factual information to squelch it.

I have had the experience of trying to run groups of expectant mothers, which I wrote up a number of years ago in *Mental Hygiene* (Caplan, 1951), in which I used a different approach. I encouraged mothers to talk. I had some nurses sitting in with me, and after an hour's session with the expectant mothers, I used to have to spend about an hour and a half with the nurses to deal with their anxieties. They felt that I was doing something terribly, terribly dangerous. Because I am of course used to handling irrational material, it did not upset me, but it upset the nurses tremendously. So I suppose that if you want to run classes for expectant mothers with nurses who have not been extensively trained to deal with irrational material without discomfort, then the only way to do it is by structuring the situation so that the irrational material does not come out.

There is one other point. Usually when I talk in these terms to an audience in which there are women, some of whom have had babies, I see on their faces expressions of disbelief. They say, 'Well, this is a psychiatrist who likes to play around with unconscious material and he imagines that it is there or else he stimulates it.'

Women who have had babies can look back and remember their pregnancy and say, 'This never happened to me. I do not believe it.' The reason for this is very interesting. They say it because the change in equilibrium between ego and id, which starts around about the end of the first trimester, and continues to about two or three weeks post-partum, then changes back to its previous state. The situation returns to normal, and there is a complete and massive repression of all those ideas and fantasies which the woman voiced during pregnancy. Four weeks later she has forgotten them, just as she has forgotten the fantasies and conflicts of early childhood and adolescence. The same kind of repressing mechanism takes over; and if you speak to her at that time she does not remember that she said any of these things to you.

I have one very good example, which I quoted in my *Concepts of Mental Health and Consultation* (1959), of a patient whom I analysed all the way through pregnancy, and then saw three weeks later. She acted as though she had forgotten completely all the things we had been talking about during pregnancy, all the fantasies that she had had about how she was going to give birth to a monster, how her milk would be sour, and how she had damaged her womanhood, and so on. It was quite a hard job to say to her, 'Now look here, Mrs. Smith, don't you remember that six weeks ago we talked about this or that?' and she said, 'No, I don't remember a thing about it.' It was possible in her case to revive these memories. This was of great importance because she had fantasied beforehand that she was going to give birth to a monster; and the poor girl gave birth to a baby with multiple congenital abnormalities; and the baby died. Her reaction was, 'This is what I had coming to me. Reality has confirmed my fantasies. All the time you said they were only fantasies, but they were not fantasies, they were true. I did give birth to a monster.' And then it was necessary for us to discuss the fact that this was not a monster, but a baby with congenital abnormalities, and her fantasies were based upon conflicts which we had discussed at length; and the fact that she gave birth to a baby with congenital abnormalities was a coincidence and did not prove that God was punishing her. We were able in that case to uncover a situation which probably occurs very often, but which is usually completely concealed. In the case of a woman whose child dies, or who gives birth to a crippled child, you do not notice that area at all. She does not know about it because it is all suppressed; but it is there under the surface causing her to feel guilty and that this is a punishment for her sins.

The important aspects of this change of equilibrium of ego and id are the following. First, that although there is relatively little arousal of anxiety when this material comes to the surface, compared with what there would be with the woman in her normal state of mind, there is, nevertheless, some. This anxiety is of a free-floating nature, that is to say, the woman is generally anxious. Later, in many women the anxiety becomes fixed to some particular idea or situation; and that is why phobias are so common in pregnancy. 'I mustn't look at a mouse; I mustn't see a rat; I mustn't look at an ugly man; if I don't have grapes when I ask for them my baby will be born with a birthmark,' and so on; not to mention all those irrational fears: that she will die during delivery; that her milk will be out of order; that the baby will be deformed, and so on. If you consider the themes of these phobias you will notice that many of them have a self-punishing character: that the woman is going to die, that her sexual apparatus is damaged, that the baby will be damaged, and so on. I suppose that some of you have heard, I was going to say the 'old wives' tale', but it is not an 'old wives' tale', it is an 'old obstetrician's tale', that the smile of the Mona Lisa is the smile of a woman who has just given birth, and is looking at her baby and discovering that it is not deformed. She is smiling because she has given birth to a healthy baby. As a matter of fact, many obstetricians will say that one of the first questions a mother asks after delivery is, 'Is the baby all right?' And one of the first things many wise obstetricians do is to show the mother the baby and to tell her, 'He has all his fingers and toes.' And what the woman is very interested in is not only the fingers and toes, especially if it is a male baby.

So the implication in the content of these pregnancy fears is that some damage will be visited upon the mother or upon the baby; and if you listen to the fantasies, you discover that the content of the fears is directly related to the feelings of guilt the woman had in regard either to conflicts with her mother or to masturbation. Behind these conflicts lie her ambivalent mixed feelings about her sexual functioning.

If this is the origin of these fears, it will not accomplish much to reassure her on a factual basis. You may give her the reassurance that the chances of having a deformed baby are very small and that the number of women who die during labour nowadays is minimal. These are reality stories, but they do not seem to convince these women. They keep on having the fears afterwards, although they may subsequently hide them from the obstetrician and from the nurse, because they feel that after they have been told the reality situation, there must be something peculiar about them if they are still worrying about it. You can make use of this knowledge by letting the expectant mother know that you realize that she still has this fear even though you have reassured her. You can say, 'We really do not know fully what these fears are due to, and although I am telling you the truth, you are not going to believe me 100 per cent.'

That is one aspect of the problem, but the other aspect of it is probably more important, namely, that as these old conflicts are revived during pregnancy, there is now a chance of a new solution. The new solution which we want to avoid is that the woman will begin to solve her problems about sexual damage, about guilt in her relations with her mother, or about jealousy of her sister, etc., by involving the future baby in the solution. The baby may then come, for example, to mean to her the damaged part of herself. Even though, when the baby is born, she sees that he is not damaged, underneath she may still have some fear that he is. This is one of the factors responsible for the not unusual picture of the woman who shops around from doctor to doctor thinking that there is something wrong with her baby. Everyone says there is nothing wrong, and so she goes to someone else. And the cause very often is that she is convinced that there is something wrong with the baby, based upon the fact that during pregnancy she revived some fantasies of guilt, and then said to herself, as it were, 'There is no doubt that my baby will be born defective because of this. This will be my cross which I will have to carry for the rest of my life.' And when the baby is born, the baby becomes part of the whole problem which she is working out in this way. She punishes herself by carrying the cross of a disordered baby. One of the reasons that she shops around is that, if someone finds something wrong with the baby, she will feel reassured; because whatever he finds wrong will be minor compared with the fantasy crippling which she felt was bound to occur to this child.

Another example is the woman who had old problems of jealousy of a younger sister which she was not able to deal with adequately. As she revives these problems, she may begin to worry that she will give birth to a girl. She does not connect these two thoughts and you will find that the eighth month is about the time when this particular sibling-jealousy problem comes to the surface. Incidentally, we need a good deal more work to investigate what are the time relations of the emergence of various problems in pregnant women. I have the feeling, and it has still to be confirmed by future work, that there is an orderly sequence of emergence of themes. About the middle of the pregnancy, conflicts with the mother come to the surface; and later on, masturbatory difficulties emerge; and quite late on, sibling-rivalry conflicts come to the surface. Why this is, or whether it is true or not, I do not know; but this represents an impression based on my experience.

Anyway, round about the eighth month I found one particular girl who began to say, 'I have a feeling that my baby is going to be a girl, and I am a bit worried about this. I would like it to be a boy.' And at the same time she was telling me about some fantasies, or memories, of her old conflicts with her sister; how jealous she had felt, and how she had wanted to push her sister down the stairs. She told me that she had broken her sister's leg on one occasion. I do not know whether it was true or imagined that she had done this damage. She was talking about the baby being a girl and, at the same time, she was worrying whether she would be a good mother or not. As I put all these items together, I got what appeared to be the story, that she felt that her baby was going to be a girl, and her baby would be representative nowadays of her sister, and she would damage the baby as she had

84

done her sister; and this would be the punishment for her having damaged her sister. Now if, in fact, a girl like that does give birth to a female child, there is the danger that her relationship with that child will not be the untrammelled relationship of an ordinary mother to her baby, with the baby being defined in its own right. The danger will be that she will perceive and treat that baby as the present embodiment of her sister.

The important point is to be able to spot these kinds of situation, and if necessary, to do what I did in that particular case. I pointed out to the woman that her old problems with her sister, whatever had happened, were over and done with; and that this was a new baby which had nothing whatever to do with her sister. It was not her sister, and it was not a representative of her sister. It was going to be a new baby. It might be a girl, or it might be a boy; but whether it was a girl or whether it was a boy, it would still be an individual in its own right. It was not inevitable that she would continue with this new person the conflict which she had had with another person, namely, with her sister.

This particular type of case needs to be dealt with by a mental health specialist. On the other hand, I think that it is possible during pregnancy for nurses and obstetricians to be on the lookout for particularly strong manifestations of this kind of material, and where they identify such a case to refer it at that stage. It usually takes only a couple of sessions for a psychiatrist to handle such a case at that particular stage. If it is allowed to continue and leads to a disturbed mother-child relationship, the latter can usually not be spotted until it results in a disturbance in the child. This may then necessitate two or three years of psychiatric work with the sick child.

In addition to this I believe that it is possible to think in terms of obstetricians and nurses educating the pregnant woman to realize that when the baby comes along it will be an individual in its own right, separate and different from everyone else she has dealt with in her life in the past. It is not the embodiment of her sister, or of her father, or of her mother. It is not a symbol of sex, or of a damaged sexual apparatus. It is not a cross to bear. It is

85

none of these things. It is a baby, an individual, a human being, and she has to build up a relationship with it on these reality grounds. Such education would tend to counteract stereotyping perceptions if the predisposing forces were not too powerful.

Attitude to the Future Baby

Now I come to the material dealing more definitely with the relationship to the future baby. This is described in my book *Concepts of Mental Health and Consultation,* and I shall not therefore go into it here in very great detail. As you remember from your reading, there are three areas that you can scan during pregnancy which will give you information about the kind of relationship which the woman will have with her baby immediately after its birth. It will not give you the power to predict exactly what kind of mother-child relationship there will be, because the mother-child relationship, as we shall discuss in the next chapter, is a circular process involving two people, each of whom is making a contribution to it. It does not just come from the mother. The kind of baby, the sex of the baby, the appearance of the baby, the reaction pattern of the baby, all these kinds of things, which no one can predict in advance, will influence how the mother will feel towards it. But you can predict what the mother is going to feed into the mother-child relationship, by listening to how the mother talks about three different topics during pregnancy.

First, what is her attitude towards conception and towards the pregnancy itself? I mention this in order to dismiss it, because as far as I can make out there is very little correlation between how the expectant mother felt when she became pregnant, or feels now about the pregnancy, and her future attitude to her baby. Women who initially reject their pregnancy with a viciousness, and with a power, and with a passion, which sometimes upset their medical and nursing attendants, may have as good a chance as anyone else of having a healthy relationship to their babies. As we know, a large proportion, especially of primiparae in our urban culture, are quite upset when they become pregnant. It upsets their career plans. In any case pregnancy is uncomfortable, yet they are supposed to like being pregnant, and no one has much sympathy for them if they do not like the idea of becoming pregnant. It is supposed to be the goal and the role of every married woman to become pregnant, and yet they do not like the idea. They do not like the early feeling of sickness, and so on. They feel miserable at the beginning; and right at the end of pregnancy they feel just as miserable. The obstetricians certainly know more about this than I do, but I think there is a peak of feeling bad at the beginning, and then it dies off and they feel well, and another little hump further on when they feel that this is going to go on for ever, and they say, 'How much longer am I going to go on wearing these same lousy old maternity dresses, and looking like a slob?' You are all familiar with this. Now this misery about the pregnancy, and about the interruption in their normal life, is not related to the development of the relationship to the baby, because I do not believe that when they are talking this way they are talking about a baby. They are talking about pregnancy. They are talking about conception. They are talking about the interference with their lives. They are not talking about the baby that will come.

Incidentally, I do not believe that the nausea and the vomiting of early pregnancy are psychosomatic. Surely a woman who vomits feels sick, and surely a woman in the early stages of pregnancy may be rejecting the pregnancy at the same time as she vomits, and that makes her reject the pregnancy even more. Psycho-analysts can, out of their own imagination, conjure up a whole host of fantasies of the connection between a woman rejecting her pregnancy and vomiting the whole time. This may mean, for example, that she is vomiting out the baby, that she is rejecting the baby by spewing it out in vomit. All I can say is that none of the cases that I have seen shows any evidence that the nausea and vomiting have a strong psychogenic element, except the cases of hyperemesis gravidarum; and I think those are quite different. In those cases where the women, if you let them, would vomit themselves to death, you almost invariably find women with very disturbed personalities who in the past have dealt with other difficulties in life through disorders of the gastro-intestinal tract.

G
87

These are quite different from the ordinary nausea and vomiting cases in early pregnancy.

I would just point out one fallacy which I have already mentioned in my book, and that is that some people say this condition is psychogenic because you can very often remove the symptom by psychological means. You can hypnotize the woman and stop her vomiting, or you can use suggestion. When my wife was feeling sick in her pregnancy and we were in a little town in England, we went to the local doctor, and he gave her a bottle of medicine. And he took me on one side (I was a very young physician) and he said, 'Doctor, I just want to let you know the important thing about this medicine is that it's coloured red. That red is a very useful colour. You will laugh at me, but red is a very potent colour; and when you want to give some good medicine, make it red.' It did not stop her vomiting; but maybe that was because she was the wife of a psychiatrist, and I unfortunately, when we came away, made some remarks about my colleague's liking for the colour red, so maybe I undid his magic. But the point is that, even though you can relieve a symptom by suggestion, by psychological means, this is no proof at all that psychological factors have been important in the aetiology. After all, you can remove the pain of an inoperable carcinoma by hypnotism. Pain does have a final common path which is in the psychological sphere, and you can interrupt it at that level. You can exert a psychosomatic effect on a somatic symptom.

Let us now proceed to the two areas that are important in the development of the mother-child relationship. First of all we will discuss the attitude towards the foetus. You are all familiar with this. If you allow an expectant mother to talk to you about her foetus, you will get quite an interesting story that is characteristic for that particular woman. A group of women can be distributed on a gradient scale in regard to how they relate to their foetus. At one end of the scale are women who regard the foetus in a purely intellectual way; they understand that it is growing inside them; they can feel it as a lump, and that is all. If you ask, 'Have you got any feelings about it?', they will answer, 'No. Who can have feelings about something like that? Do I have feelings about my stomach, or about my kidneys, or about my spleen? These are things inside me. I can sometimes feel that the foetus protrudes. I can feel that it is getting bigger. But this is not a thing that one has feelings about.' At the other end of the scale are women who talk about the foetus from the beginning as though it were a little human being. They endow it with human characteristics. They know where its head is, where its arms are, where its bottom is, and where its legs are. They pay attention to its movements; and they play with it; and they have feelings about it; and they may love it. The love of a woman, at the extreme end of the scale, for her foetus is a very intense and very definite feeling. She gives the foetus a name, and she gives it a sex. The latter varies, some women are not certain and they give it two sexes. They say, 'If it is a boy it is called Peter, if it is a girl it is called Mary.' They play with it, and they try and involve their husbands in the games. The husbands sometimes like this, and sometimes they worry about it. The attitude of the husband to the foetus may not be the same as the attitude of his wife. I remember one woman who was very fond of her foetus, but when I spoke to the husband he said, 'That little blighter, he's already kicking me out of bed.'

There is another parameter which intersects this scale, and that is the type of feelings about the foetus, because a woman may endow the foetus with vivid human characteristics and yet have negative feelings towards it. Some women already during pregnancy, as they talk about their foetus, can be seen to have very mixed feelings about it. You can hear them telling you almost openly what they are going to feel about the baby when it comes. They say, 'This is a burden. When I am sitting reading the newspaper, this damn little thing suddenly kicks the paper away from me. I can't sleep on my stomach as I always used to. It gets in the way. It wakens me up at night.' As they talk about it you hear an acid tone, and a bell should ring in your mind, 'Watch out for trouble.'

There appears to be a relationship between the grouping of women at these two poles, and the time-lag between when the baby is born and when the mother develops what David Levy has called 'full maternal feeling'. As you know, sometimes it takes a few hours, sometimes a few days, and sometimes a few weeks, for a mother who has given birth to a baby to get a rush of maternal feeling, a feeling that 'This is my baby, and I love him, and I don't care what he looks like, and I don't care what anyone says, this is the most beautiful baby in the world'; this feeling of intense, warm protectiveness and sympathy which is the maternal feeling. You can predict this time-lag by paying attention to the attitude towards the foetus. The nearer the woman is to the intellectual, objective pole, the longer will be the time-lag, other things being equal. Other things are seldom equal. There are other factors which influence the time-lag. But this is one important factor. The more intense the relationship, and the more the expectant mother personifies the foetus, the shorter will be the time-lag after the baby is born. In fact, in certain extreme cases, there is no time-lag at all; and the woman continues to have the relationship to the baby that she had to the foetus, interrupted only by the mechanics of delivery. If she had an anaesthetic, there will be some little time-lag. If she herself was present, as it were, while the baby was being born, then the feeling continues straight through. If you talk to such women about their newborn babies, they will talk in the same terms about the baby as they did about the foetus. If you say to them, 'How is it that you feel this way already about your baby?', they will say, 'Well, I feel this way, because after all, I've been carrying him all this time, and it's the same person isn't it, now he's outside. Before he was inside, but he is the same person. I just have the same feelings.' For the women at the other pole of the scale, when the baby is born it is a new individual, and they have to develop a relationship to it. We shall talk more about this in the next chapter. There are advantages and disadvantages in both groups.

The last area that you would scan in order to be able to predict something about the attitude of the woman to her newborn baby, is in regard to what the woman says about her fantasies about the baby-to-be. Fantasies about the baby-to-be can usually be separated quite easily from the woman's feelings about her foetus. Not all women, but many women, will have night-dreams and day-dreams, and imaginations, and thoughts, and plans about what kind of a baby they are going to have, and what is going to happen to the baby. If you take the time to listen, and to ask her a few questions about it, you will get stories from the expectant mother which will give you a characteristic feel for the psychological preparation she is making for the coming baby. You will find many women who will have fantasies about babies of all different ages. They will fantasy the baby when it is just born; and when it is small; and when it has grown a bit bigger; and as a toddler; and they will think about it in the distant future. Their fantasies vary from time to time. They may imagine babies of both sexes, and they usually do not know quite what the baby is going to be, how he is going to look, and where he is going to go. When they think about the baby as a small baby, they imagine themselves being very happy with it, and feeding it, and washing it, and dressing it up nicely. There are all kinds of different fantasies. That is the characteristic healthy picture.

You can get variations on the healthy picture, and you can get unhealthy pictures. By unhealthy pictures, I mean the kind of pictures from which you would predict difficulty. First of all, you will find women who in their fantasies can never imagine their baby as an infant. They can never imagine it as a youngster of less than three or four months old. It is as though this particular area has been blotted out. Almost invariably when you find that situation, if you ask them a few questions, you discover that these women are worried by a small baby. They are afraid that they will break it, or damage it, or that they will be unable to take care of it. They have never had a baby before. They remember seeing children, but they have never held a small baby. 'How do you hold a small baby; when you're bathing it, doesn't it slide down when you put soap on it? Doesn't it slide down into the water and get drowned?' 'Their necks are very tender, and maybe I will twist its neck.' All their talk about small babies is about very frightening happenings.

These women are telling you, as well as they can, 'I am going to have difficulty with my baby from birth to about two or three months.' There are some women who are always talking about their children at college age, or later on; and as you listen to them talking like this, they seem to be talking about their children almost as direct representatives of themselves. As you listen to the stories, you get an uncanny feeling that the baby is already being cast rather rigidly into a special role; and the details of this role are designed to make up for what the parent could not do when she was younger. The girl who wanted to be a ballet dancer and could not manage it, fantasies her baby becoming a very famous ballerina. A woman who wanted to go on to college and could not, fantasies her child as being a university graduate and receiving his degree. The girl who wanted to be a boy, fantasies having a boy who has what she did not have.

This is a danger signal again, but of a somewhat different kind; because it tells you that this expectant mother is expecting a baby who will be used by her to solve one of her own problems. You are seeing here the beginning of a characteristic picture of a disturbance of mother-child relationships, where the mother does not perceive the child as he is, and does not allow the child to be as he is, but moulds him right along to fit into a quite definite prescription which has special meaning to her.

You can also be alert to this if you find someone who always fantasies a boy, or always fantasies a girl. The child is never anything else – always a boy, or always a girl. In such a case it is a good idea to take a closer look and to ask why it is inevitable for her that she should have a boy or a girl. Of course, if someone is so set on a boy in fantasy in this way, if the baby turns out to be a boy then the danger is it is going to be pushed in certain predetermined directions, and if it is a girl there is likely to be an overly disappointed reaction; and the baby may be rejected. You have to be very careful about the culture in considering the meaning of this, since in certain cultures most mothers want a boy because boys are the only people who count, and girls are of no importance. Whether the mother is a queen who has to have an heir to the throne, or a more lowly citizen, if the child is born a girl she is likely to be a little rejected in these cultures.

There is one other aspect of these fantasies about the baby-to-be. If a woman fantasies very strongly a certain kind of baby, and she is quite specific about what the baby is going to be like, when the baby is born you may have a falling-in-love phenomenon, an infatuation phenomenon. By an infatuation phenomenon I mean that, when the woman first sees the baby, she does not in fact perceive him as he is but she 'clicks' him into place into her pre-existing fantasy. So she falls in love not with this baby that others can see, but with a baby that she imagines she sees. It is not this baby at all, it is the fantasy she has been carrying around within her for several months.

This is what happens in infatuations in grown-up people. I suppose many of my readers have experienced this. This is falling in love at first sight. You suddenly know that this is your predetermined soulmate, or whatever word you want to use; and he is marvellous, he is wonderful, and everything that you could ever have wished. You always imagined that you would meet such a person; and if, sometimes unfortunately on the basis only of this, you marry him, you may find that after several months or several years there is a falling-out-of-love phenomenon, when you discover to your great surprise and to your tremendous disappointment, that this person is not at all the person that you saw before. You never were seeing this person before.

There is some of this misperception in all love relationships, hence the popular saying, 'Love is blind.' When you love someone, the loving relationship inevitably has some element of not seeing the person as he is but of projecting from inside yourself some ideal image you have been carrying around with you.

The danger for the woman who becomes infatuated with her infant is the danger (a) that she will not perceive his needs, and (b) that she may fall out of love; and she may fall out of love very often round about the eighth or ninth month of his life, which will lead to great difficulties. As he begins to exercise his own independence, he may take a step or two out of her picture, to such an extent that the picture is rudely shattered. This may lead to a massive kind of rejection of the child who has previously been an angel and everything marvellous that there could be in heaven and earth.

93

Effects on Husband and Children

Before I end this chapter I wish to refer briefly to one more theme which is of great importance to our work, namely, the importance of pregnancy for the husband and for the rest of the family. I think that I have already given sufficient data upon which we can build up a fair conception of the effect on the husband of his wife's increasing irritability, of her demanding instead of giving, and of her change in sexual appetite. The husband of the pregnant woman has a very difficult role especially in our present-day culture. In our culture husbands are not held in high esteem during pregnancy and delivery. Some people have attempted to remedy this by involving the husband actively in taking care of his pregnant wife and enlisting his collaboration in the delivery process. This is all to the good, as long as they do not push him too far, and expect from him more than certain husbands are able to do. I think we should always be aware of the dangers of mass production in our work. The idea that all husbands have to take part in their wife's delivery is sometimes taking things a bit too far. Some husbands just cannot do this; and if you push them into it, you make delivery a burden to them. You do not enhance their feelings of self-respect, which are usually wounded by all the jokes that are made about the husbands of pregnant women, and especially about the husbands of women in delivery. There are funny stories about the poor fellow who is walking up and down outside, and they come and tell him, 'You've had twins [or triplets].' The expectant father is mostly a figure of ridicule in our culture.

This is extremely unfortunate, because from what I have been saying it is clear that he should have an important role in providing emotional supplies for his wife. He should be making sure that her 'battery is charged up' so that she can afterwards help her child. He has the task of giving her support during the crises of pregnancy so that her weakened ego can be strengthened by his.

Not only the husband, but also the other children are apt to be quite upset during pregnancy. First of all, they are upset by the

94

woman's introversion. She withdraws interest from her surroundings, and this includes her interest in them. Especially at the beginning of pregnancy when she is upset and may be vomiting, and feels depressed, and has sudden mood swings, the other children cannot understand what is happening to her. All they know is that mother has changed; and a small child who feels that mother has changed reacts to this usually by becoming more demanding; so there is a vicious circle. The child becomes more demanding; the woman just cannot bear him; and she moves further away to get a bit of a rest; so he feels more deprived, and he becomes more demanding; and so it goes on.

The husband may also be upset; and in our culture this may lead to the beginnings of marital disharmony. This is especially so because of the changes in the wife's sexual appetite, if this happens to be a change for the worse. She becomes frigid and loses her desire; and at the same time she becomes irritable and sensitive and easily insulted. In these circumstances, if the husband does not understand what is going on, he is apt to feel that she no longer loves him, he may ascribe this to his having made her pregnant, especially in view of her possible initial negative reaction to conception. He is apt to be quite sexually frustrated too, and either to have fantasies of infidelity or to go out and look for alternative satisfaction. Sometimes marriages begin to break up on this particular rock.

REFERENCES

CAPLAN, GERALD (1951). 'Mental Hygiene Work with Expectant Mothers.' *Ment. Hygiene*, **35**, 41.

CAPLAN, GERALD (1959). *Concepts of Mental Health and Consultation*. Washington, D.C.: Children's Bureau Publication No. 373.

CHAPTER 4

Early Mother-Child Relationships and the Effects of Mother-Child Separation

DEVELOPMENT OF THE MOTHER-CHILD RELATIONSHIP

ONE of the most important insights achieved in recent years is our recognition of the importance of the emotional milieu as a critical factor in the child's total development. The quality of the emotional interplay in the family circle not only has a potent effect on the child's emotional unfolding, it also exerts a great influence on his capacity to make use of his intellectual endowment, and it influences his general physical growth and development.

During the first year of life, the effects of the family on the child are conveyed almost entirely via the mother. Her relationship with him is his key to the social world. She is the first 'other' in his awareness. Through his relationship with this other person, he takes the first step in developing the recognition of his own self-identity, which is the basis for all his subsequent personality development. It is a paradox that the baby's awareness of himself comes as a secondary step after the baby's awareness that there is someone outside himself. There is a well-known theory that the baby's awareness of himself comes first through his mouth, through his relationship with the nipple, whether it is the nipple of the bottle or the nipple of the mother's breast. This nipple comes and goes; and since it is sometimes there and sometimes not there, the baby begins to realize that there is something which is apart from himself. When he realizes that there is an 'other' in the world, that implies also the recognition of himself as an entity separate from the 'other'.

The emotional atmosphere in the day-to-day happenings in the family circle affects the mother's relationship with her child. This is the channel through which they impinge upon him in a significant way. I shall deal in Chapter 5 with the emotional effect of the family on the mental health of its members, including the child; but in the first year of life what goes on in the family affects the child through affecting the mother.

Towards the end of the first year, the child begins to develop relationships not only with his mother but also with his father; and during the second year with his siblings and other family members. To begin with, these new links are patterned by him along the lines of his primary bond with his mother. It is not until many years later that other people are perceived and dealt with in their own right and are not connected in some way with the mother and the family. It is as though the child tunes into the social world on the 'mother-child relationship wavelength', and ever afterwards his perception of messages from the outside world is coloured, or moulded, by that particular wavelength.

In thinking about the mother-child relationship, it is important to realize that this is a relationship between *two people,* even when in early infancy one of these people has no recognizable personality. It is hard to think of a newborn infant as a person because he is different in many ways from our concept of a person; and yet the relationship of the mother and child must always be conceived of as a relationship of two active units. Even when the baby is first born, he does have some individuality which is expressed in his physical shape and appearance, and in the sensitivity of his reactions to stimuli, as well as in his general pattern of response in regard to activity and passivity. Margaret Fries of New York has done some interesting work in testing the differences among the reaction patterns of different infants. She drops a weight which makes a loud noise near the infant, and then times how long it takes before he jumps and what kind of a jump he gives. She finds that babies can be fairly easily divided into two extreme groups of those who jump a lot and jump quickly, and those who jump little and slowly. As you would expect, there is also an intermediate group. Incidentally, many of you may know of the work of Sontag of Yellow Springs, Ohio. He has done the same kind of thing with foetuses, by banging a big tuning fork and putting it on the expectant mother's abdomen and then ascertaining the change in the heart rate of the foetus, and change in the foetal movements. He finds that foetuses have a fairly consistent pattern of reactions.

Although these phenomena, the baby's shape and appearance and reaction-time and sensitivity, are not consciously intended by the baby as communications, as messages which he is sending to the mother, they are nevertheless received by the mother and reacted to by her almost as though they were. Her own behaviour to the baby is modified by them. Her behaviour in turn affects the baby's reaction. So that the interchange between the mother and the child must be conceived of as a circular system which is in constant dynamic flux. It is, in effect, a reverberating circular system. The messages coming from one person produce an effect on the other. New messages from the latter then change the first, and so on. The whole system is in circular reverberating movement. So we have to take great care when we call it a 'mother-child relationship' that we are not misled into conceiving of it as an unidirectional flow, as something that comes from the mother and goes to the child; and which has consistency of its own, which is not being constantly influenced by the actual interchange between the mother and the child, and the child and the mother. We sometimes invent words for things and then get misled by our own words.

It is also important to realize that although there is some over-all stability of the patterning of this relationship, which is dependent on the mother's more or less unchanging personality, the child, who is the other element of the equation, is in a state of continuous developmental change, especially marked in his earliest years. A child is not a little adult. He passes through successive phases of development which are qualitatively different from the adult state. This means that over a time continuum of months or years the mother-child relationship must be expected to show parallel successive changes in its pattern.

The mother-child relationship must be expected to change as the child changes because the whole system is bound to change if one element in it is changing. In practice this is found to be true. A mother who may feel happy and relaxed in her relationship to her child at one stage of his development, may experience tension and difficulties at a successive stage for a variety of reasons. These may include not only the involvement of this relationship in other emotional problems at that time, but also the revival in her of unsolved problems from her childhood in her relationship with her own mother, stimulated by her day-to-day contact with the manifestations of the same phase of development in her child. Thus, a mother may feel quite secure in handling her baby's feeding problems, but when she begins to deal with toilet-training this may stimulate and revive unresolved difficulties from her childhood battles with her own mother in this regard. This is one of the reasons why I said in Chapter 3 that you cannot predict during pregnancy what the mother-child relationship is going to be. You can only predict what the mother introduces into the circular reverberating system; although this is very important.

When a mother is dealing with the toilet-training of her child, the intimate relationship with the child engaged in toilet-training battles with her may stimulate old memories of her battles with her mother at that particular stage, and this may upset her management of the child. On the other hand, just as we said in regard to pregnancy, when old problems are revived there is the possibility of new and better solutions. You find that certain mothers have a personality maturation which occurs in quite a spontaneous manner during their mothering. Going back to the example I have just given, a girl who had difficulties in regard to toilet-training herself may never have resolved them appropriately. These problems are then revived when she becomes a mother and engages in toilet-training with her own child. She now has the possibility as an adult of overcoming these old problems as she deals with them in regard to her child.

The same principle applies, for instance, to people dealing with difficulties in their professional work, to which they may have become especially sensitive because of personal life problems from the past. If they have these problems, it may mean that they may have special difficulty in handling the present situation. But if they are able to overcome the difficulty and deal with the present situation, they themselves are likely to show personality maturation as a result. A question which I have often been asked is, 'What do you do as an educator if you have a student whom you recognize having difficulties with a patient because of some sensitivity in the student's own life?' One plan might be that you get the student to talk about the difficulties in his own life, and you hope that by talking with him about this you are going to be able to help him find a better solution. This will then have a general effect, and he will be better able to handle the problem of the patient. My feelings about this are quite strong. I feel that (*a*) this is unnecessary, and I will say in a moment why, and (*b*) it is undesirable because it confuses the role of the student, and it confuses the role of the educator. It turns the student into a patient, and it turns the educator into a therapist, and these are not the roles of either. Secondly, it attacks one essential goal of professional education, which is to build a professional armour and to encourage professional distance between the budding professional and the client, so that the former learns to maintain a psychological separation between his own problems and his professional tasks. Immediately you open this matter up and say to the student, 'You are having difficulties here because of some problem of your own; so now let us examine your problem', you make a hole in the armour. The implication of this is: 'When you are engaged in your professional work, this is intimately associated with the essence of your own being.' This means bringing the client very close instead of maintaining an objective distance.

It is for these reasons that I regard this method as undesirable. The reason that I regard it as unnecessary is that we find in practice that it is perfectly feasible to support the student in dealing with the problem of the patient without having to deal with his own problem in any overt manner. The only thing that you have to recognize is that the student is especially sensitive in this or that specific area; and so you need to give extra support and extra help to allow him to deal with this particular matter, which you have recognized as being especially difficult.

Now, the same kind of thing happens with a mother, and sometimes it happens spontaneously in the same way as it does with a student. The mother without any special professional help, who because of difficulties with toilet-training in her own life is having special difficulties in toilet-training her child, may on her own find ways of overcoming these difficulties and of reaching a satisfactory solution of them for her child. This success with her child means that the mother herself will no longer regard problems of dirt and control, and of putting up with society's pressures against the gratification of demands, as so difficult. This whole topic becomes for her easier and less tension-ridden than it was in the past.

This happens spontaneously sometimes, but sometimes a mother makes a mess of the toilet-training of her own child in the same way as her mother was not able to solve the problem with her. In those circumstances, if we spot this and if we are able to help her to work it out satisfactorily in her child, this has a good effect both on her and on the child without our ever having to ask her about her problems when she was a child.

In our efforts to help mothers solve their relationship problems with their children, we need to have some practical clinical yardstick with which to assess the state of the mother-child relationship at any time. This will help us to decide when to intervene, and in what degree; or when to adopt a policy of watchful inactivity while the mother makes her own attempts at solution. The important thing to realize, however, is that we must assess the relationship on the basis of our observations of what is going on currently between the mother and child, and not wait for unfortunate results in the child's development. These unfortunate results may take months or years to appear, and when they do it will probably be too late for simple remedies. You cannot therefore use disorder in a child as one of your criteria for measuring disordered mother-child relationships.

Since I conceive of the mother-child relationship as a circular reverberating system of forces altering dynamically over a time continuum and influenced constantly by developmental changes in the child as well as by changes in the emotional milieu of the family and of the social environment, it is difficult to think of a way of crystallizing it so that at any one moment in time it can be rated as healthy or unhealthy, that is to say promotive of mental health in the child or the opposite. Yet experience in well-baby centres with optimally operating mothers and healthy children, as well as clinical experience in child guidance clinics with mothers who have disturbed relationships with their children, has in the last few years provided us with a working definition of a healthy, compared with a potentially pathogenic, mother-child relationship; and this can be used as a rough guide by nurses and physicians. Allowing for all the difficulties, we can nevertheless work out a rather rough-and-ready clinical instrument. This clinical instrument depends upon a definition. I should like to define for you a healthy mother-child relationship and to contrast this with an unhealthy mother-child relationship.

A healthy mother-child relationship can be defined as one in which the mother reacts to the child *primarily* on the basis of her perception of the child's needs as a person in his own right, respect for those needs, and her attempts to satisfy them to the best of her ability, in line with the accepted practices of her culture and her society. There are four elements, (*a*) perception, (*b*) respect, (*c*) satisfaction of the child's needs, and (*d*) the child being seen as a person in his own right.

I contrast this with the definition of an unhealthy, or potentially pathogenic relationship in which the mother perceives and reacts to her child *primarily* on the basis of her own needs, and her attempts to satisfy these by means of her behaviour through the child. The child is not perceived by her as a person in his own right; and even if he is occasionally so perceived, his needs are not respected; and certainly, of course, his needs are not satisfied.

Now clearly, this definition is not independent of culture. Cultural factors are introduced explicitly into the definition; but in addition to that, the perception of a child as a person in his own right whose needs are worthy of respect may not fit into the value or role pattern of certain societies. There are certain societies where children are not supposed to have separate individuality, or to have needs in their own right; and therefore, a mother in such a society would not perceive the child in this way. Her society defines a child as something different. But in regard to our culture of the present day, the definition seems to hold from this point of view.

You will notice that as I stated the definitions both of healthy and of unhealthy relationships, I accented the word 'primarily'. A healthy mother-child relationship involves reciprocal gratification of mother and child. The mother certainly satisfies her own needs to be motherly, to be protecting, to be nurturing, and to be comforting when she relates to her baby. In fact, one of the signs of a healthy mother-child relationship is a mother who herself gets a tremendous satisfaction from respecting and satisfying the needs of her child. You would be suspicious of a mother-child relationship if the mother were not herself getting obvious satisfaction in the process. But the goal of these needs is the baby's welfare; and the mother's gratification is consequent upon the satisfaction of the baby's wishes. This is to be contrasted with an unhealthy relationship where the mother uses the child for gratification of non-motherly needs in herself, such as personal ambition, need to be loved, solution of problems of marital disharmony, and so on.

Just to make this definition more realistic and to give it a less abstract feel, I shall contrast two situations. In both of them, a mother is standing in the kitchen ironing clothes, and her two-and-a-half-year-old little boy is on the floor of the kitchen, playing with blocks, building a tower.

In one case, the mother is ironing and the little boy builds his tower of blocks, and somehow the tower does not stand up. It keeps falling down, as towers sometimes do; and the child gets more and more frustrated, and becomes more and more tense. He just cannot manage to build his tower; it keeps toppling down. The mother is doing her ironing, but out of the corner of her eye she sees the child in his play, and she notices that the child is just about to start weeping with frustration. So she interrupts her ironing and she turns to the child, and she picks him up and she hugs him and kisses him and tells him that mother loves him, and she kneels down and she helps him to build a tower that will stand up. This is a healthy mother-child relationship, or rather, it is one sign of a healthy mother-child relationship; you cannot make an assessment on the basis of just one incident. But here you see a conflict between the needs of this mother and her child. She has a big pile of ironing to do, she has to get on with her work, and yet she perceives the needs of the child, and she puts aside her own needs in order to attend to his. When he required comfort and support and help, she put aside her ironing, and she went and helped him.

In contrast here is another picture. While the mother is ironing, she is thinking how miserable she is because her husband, who is a commercial traveller, has been away now for three days, and she is feeling quite lonely and depressed. She has all this ironing to do and she says to herself, 'What do I do all day long but just wash and iron and stick in the kitchen, while he is off gallivanting around, and goodness knows what he is up to!' Meanwhile her child is there on the kitchen floor, and he is building towers; and his towers are lovely. He is feeling very full of success in his building. And suddenly the woman's feeling of loneliness and misery causes her to stop ironing. She puts down the iron, and she takes the little child and she lifts him up from the game, and she hugs him and kisses him, and tells him how much she loves him, and how much he loves her. And the child is as frustrated as the dickens because his game has been interrupted, and his activity in which he was so successfully engaged has been set aside.

Now here you see superficially the same situation, but there is a tremendous difference. The second woman lifted the child up and hugged him and kissed him because she was herself in need of love and comfort and affection, not because she perceived this need in the child. She interrupted the child's game, and she did not do this on the basis of her perception of the child's need at all, but she was using the child as an instrument for the gratification of her own needs, and to relieve her own misery. You would not say merely on the basis of this that this is an unhealthy relationship, but the fact is that this is a rather important piece of evidence to which you would give serious weight in deciding the nature of the link between that mother and child.

It is important to note that the definition of a healthy mother-child relationship, which is based on the mother's perception of the child as an individual in his own right, implies the psychological separation of the child from the mother. During the past few years we have been very much impressed by evidence, to be presented in the second part of this chapter, regarding the harmful effects of prolonged geographical separation of a child from his mother during the first few years of life; harmful effects on the child, and incidentally on the mother. Such deprivation of maternal care interferes significantly with the personality development of the child. It is, therefore, a little difficult to realize that a certain degree of psychological separation of mother and child is essential to healthy development.

In this connection, it is well to remember that although physical separation between mother and child occurs when the umbilical cord is cut, in many cases psychological separation does not occur at the same time. You will remember that in Chapter 3 I talked about certain expectant mothers who develop relationships of varying intensity to the foetus, and to fantasied babies which may equally be part of themselves. The baby after birth may inherit these relationships. In these cases, the earliest stages of mother-child relationships are in large part *symbiotic,* that is to say, the mother is relating to the child symbolically as though it were part of herself. After all, the foetus is part of herself. The fact that she endows it with personality does not separate it from herself. When the foetus comes out and becomes a baby, if the relationship continues as before, the mother is relating to the baby as though to herself. We see two people, but to that mother it is herself to whom she is relating. She identifies the baby with herself, and she identifies herself with the baby. This means that she is very sensitive to the expression of the baby's needs which she experiences, as it were, subjectively rather than by objective perception. This is especially noticeable in the successful breast-feeding situation, and as I mentioned above, when you watch such a mother breast-feeding her baby it looks as though you are seeing a unity. The mother does not have to look at the baby to know what the baby is feeling; she feels it as though it were one of her own limbs.

This attitude on the part of the mother towards the child as a psychological extension of herself during the early weeks or months of life is mirrored by a lack of differentiation of the feeling of self in the child. As much as we can imagine what a young infant feels, he probably does not feel himself as a separate person. The vague feeling that we imagine he has is a sort of universal feeling. It takes a young child about three to five months before he is able to recognize the mother as a separate person; and until he recognizes her as a separate person, he cannot recognize himself as a separate person.

Over these months differentiation in the child should take place, but it is essential, in order for the differentiation of otherness and selfness in the child to develop, that the mother's attitude and relationship to the child should also change during this period. If the mother continues to relate to the child as an extension of herself, the child for his part will have difficulty in developing the concept of his own identity. This will probably lead to fundamental disorders in his personality make-up. As a matter of fact, some of the most severe psychiatric disorders of childhood, some childhood psychoses, can be traced very directly to the fact that the mother continues to relate to the child as though it were part of her own body. She continues to have a symbiotic relationship to the child, and these psychoses are called 'symbiotic psychoses', where the child has no real personality of his own, but continues, as it were, to be part and parcel of his mother.

Much research is still needed in order to chart the time relations of this basic development in mother-child relationships from the symbiotic pattern of mother-child unity to that of two separate individuals, which some people call the *anaclytic* pattern.

I do not like the word anaclytic, and I share this dislike with a famous inhabitant of Denver, namely René Spitz, who, a few years ago, when we were discussing this, suggested the term *dia-trophic*. Anaclytic means 'leaning against', and he pointed out that this word may seem to imply two structures which are leaning against each other, which may mean that the mother is leaning against the child; and indeed this can happen. He wanted to emphasize that what is involved in a healthy relationship is the child leaning against the mother, not the mother leaning against the child. What we want is a word that implies one structure supporting another, not two structures leaning against each other. Because of this he suggested the use of the word *diatrophic*. So in the group of mothers that I have been talking about, who have intense relationships with the foetus or the fantasy of the baby-to-be during pregnancy, which continue afterwards in a symbiotic unity, there must be a development from the initial symbiotic relationship to a later diatrophic relationship.

The question is, what are the time relations of this move from the original symbiotic relationship to the later diatrophic relationship? It is likely that there is a fairly wide range of individual variation in the rate of this change-over. It is usually not a sudden change; and some symbiotic features may persist into the second year, or in certain cultures much later. But in most normal cases in our culture, the change appears to start about three months after birth and to be reasonably complete before the end of the first year. There is evidence that cultural factors, particularly the educational efforts of caretaking agents such as doctors and nurses, may exert an important effect on this process; and as a matter of fact, much of parent education in well-baby clinics may be conceived of as an attempt to help the mother to 'get to know' her baby, that is to separate herself from him so that she observes his behaviour from a distance with some objectivity, in order to realize his individuality and therefore to perceive his needs.

It may be as well to emphasize that this educational process in well-baby clinics is not accomplished by giving the mother intellectual information about babies in general, although this is undoubtedly of value in other connections; but by the nurse or the doctor reporting personal observations of this baby, and affording the mother the opportunity of identifying with this procedure. Pauline Stitt, our paediatrician at the Harvard School of Public Health, is a great expert in this. If you watch her operating in a well-baby clinic, you will find that while she is carrying out her examination of the child, she is talking to the mother, and what she is saying to the mother of a young baby usually is, 'Look how he lies, look how he raises his hand. When I lift him up, see how his back goes. He is different from last week. Look at the way his eyes follow me as I move around. Now I'm putting something around his head. See how he begins to cry. It looks as though he doesn't like this cold thing. I don't know why it is that babies don't like cold things around their heads in this way. Most babies seem to cry. Notice the way he cries, and then when I take it off notice. . . .' She is carrying on a running commentary on her perceptions of the baby as a separate individual, and she is doing it in such a way that she is getting the mother to identify with her; so that, as it were, she lends her eyes and her ears to the mother to see this baby as a separate individual. And if you did not know what was happening, you would say, 'She is just talking to the mother while she's examining the child.' This is true, she is not taking any special time over it; but what she is doing is a most important aspect of well-baby clinic care. She does not do this with all mothers; but with certain mothers she does it much more than with others; and these mothers are the ones where there is, in her opinion, a delay in the development of the diatrophic relationship. What she is doing is separating the mother and child psychologically.

Such a system of promoting an optimal degree of mother-child separation has to be based on the needs of each individual case. In the majority of cases, it will not be especially needed, although it is not likely to do any harm. In certain cases, the physician or the nurse will already have been alerted during pregnancy by an especially strong relationship between the expectant mother and her foetus that she is very likely to have strongly marked symbiotic relationships with her baby. And if their observations during the early months after birth confirm this, and the pattern shows no signs of altering spontaneously as the months pass; and if efforts to separate them have been in vain, it may be advisable at the seventh or eighth month to consider referral to a psychiatrist, who will try to find out what is going on to delay so unduly the separation of the mother and the child.

On the other hand, however, I would say that this referral should come only after the nurses and the physicians have themselves made quite active efforts to encourage the separation. Most of this work can be done quite adequately by paediatricians and by nurses. This type of work is not best done by psychiatrists. Their approach would be quite different. The approach of the psychiatrist would be the much more laborious one of digging around in the personality of the mother to find out what has gone wrong there to cause her to have such an intense grasp on her baby that she cannot allow the child to be separated from her.

I wish to emphasize that what I have been saying so far applies only to certain mothers. A significant proportion of mothers do not pass through a stage of symbiotic relationship to their baby. The first relationship that they develop after the baby's birth is already a diatrophic one. These are the mothers who during pregnancy had little or no feeling towards the foetus, or who felt the foetus was a foetus, not a person. It will be recalled that in Chapter 3 we talked of women at one end of the continuum who regarded the foetus from a purely intellectual point of view as something growing inside them. Such mothers, as already mentioned, have a fairly long time lapse after the baby is born before developing maternal feeling. To these mothers, when they see their babies for the first time, the babies are little strangers, and they have to get to know them before developing a relationship, as one does with any stranger. Such women often have difficulty in understanding their baby's needs in the early stages, and this is especially so with their first babies. They consequently have more than the usual difficulty in breast-feeding, or in other early nursing procedures. Incidentally, with such mothers, the task of doctors and nurses is to reduce the psychological distance between mother and child in the first few weeks, rather than to aim at future psychological separation. Here mother and child are too far apart, and we want to bring them together.

Here again, the paediatricians and the nurses may act as models or they may encourage contact with the grandmother or a friend with well-developed maternal attitudes, with whom the young mother may identify. Referring again to Pauline Stitt : as you watch her in the well-baby clinic, you will find that with some mothers, instead of carrying on the running commentary to interpret the baby to the mother, she lifts the baby up, and she hugs it and she coos to it, and she holds it close, and she behaves in a very warm, maternal way with it. The mother watches her and identifies a little with this behaviour; at least that is the hope. In addition to that, the mother is encouraged to utilize the good efforts of warmly maternal relatives or of her mother, or her mother-in-law. The public health nurse who goes out to visit the home has a rather important task in discovering a maternal role model, and communicating with the paediatrician in the well-baby clinic, because he cannot tell from where he stands what kind of a warm maternal, or a cold non-maternal, person this relative in the home may be. What happens in these cases is that one tries to encourage the mother to have role models of warm maternal people in her relationship with the baby.

Much more active support is needed by such mothers in the early weeks, and more advice and direction in regard to details of nursing care, than in the case of mothers with symbiotic relationships. These mothers do not know what their babies feel; you have to help them feel what their babies feel, whereas with the first group you do not have to help them in that at all. They know on their own. They usually know better than you.

On the other hand, once these mothers have been helped to relate to their babies in a warm way, they usually have little trouble subsequently in allowing the children to develop toward self-differentiation, because they do not have to change from a symbiotic to a diatrophic relationship.

It may also be as well to emphasize that although a closer

relationship to the child should be actively encouraged, these mothers should not be rushed; and I just want to stress that. You have to realize that you are dealing with people who are having difficulties here. You want to help them, but you do not want to push them, and you do not want to push them especially if they show signs of special fears of small babies, which we shall discuss later. Our goal should be the development of a warm relationship by three to five months; but in cases of special difficulty, a few months longer can safely be allowed. One of the big differences between the work of the paediatrician or of the nurse in a well-baby clinic, and the work of the psychiatrist, is that the latter must achieve his goal as fast as possible. Paediatricians and nurses can take their time, they can follow the rhythm of nature, and they can often hold a watching brief in much the same way as good obstetricians.

If no satisfactory progress is made, the possibility of deeper trouble should be suspected and then they can refer the case to a psychiatrist for preventive intervention. In supervising the mother-child relationship as in other aspects of well-child care, the rhythm of development of the individual case is a prime diagnostic consideration, and this is another reason why it is important to try and arrange for continuity of care from pregnancy on; because as you can see, you can already tell during pregnancy which way some of these women are going to move. It is also very important if you can arrange to have continuity of care from one child to the next, because you begin to learn the rhythm of a particular woman in relation to her first child, and this helps in supervising the subsequent ones.

Now to summarize all this. In the first group we have a mother with very strong relationships to her foetus. Then the foetus emerges, and the umbilical cord is cut; but a psychological umbilical cord continues, and we have the situation of the symbiotic early relationship. This is perfectly healthy, but to avoid trouble it has to change to the diatrophic relationship by about three to seven months. The second polar type is the expectant mother with little or no relationship to her foetus, and then after birth this mother and her child are quite distant from each other; and our aim is to bring the two closer together as soon as possible. The problem of the paediatrician is different in these two groups of cases; in the first one he has to ensure that the symbiotic link gets undone, and the child gets psychologically separated from the mother. In the second one he has to identify that the child is too far away, and he has to bring mother and child closer together.

We have so far considered the factors influencing the mother-child relationship which originate primarily in the mother, and we now have to turn to a consideration of some factors which originate in the child. Here I am repeating some material from *Concepts of Mental Health and Consultation* (1959), in which I described the three stages in the first year of the child's life. We can divide the first year of life into three periods in relation to developmental processes in the infant which exert a major influence on the mother-child relationship.

The first period is from birth to about two to three months. The second period stretches from two to three months to about seven or eight months, and the third from about seven months to the end of the first year. This is a rough time-table, as all these time-tables must be. There are tremendous individual variations from one baby to the next, but I can say from my clinical experience that this time-table can serve as a rather useful rough-and-ready guide.

From Birth to two to three Months

The first period is characterized by the fact that the baby has no 'personality'. It is a helpless bundle of instincts, with no control over its physiological or its psychological processes, no real awareness of its environment, and no power of communication. It is completely dependent upon its mother for the maintenance of life; and although her efforts in this connection bring obvious results, the baby can give no personal thanks to the mother for her attentions. It cannot communicate with her. Many mothers, especially those who experience a well-marked maternal feeling, are positively stimulated by the helpless condition of the baby in this stage. This evokes their fullest maternal feeling. When they see the 'poor, little, helpless creature', they become comforting, nurturing, supporting, and protecting; and they derive satisfaction from the gratification of the baby's needs by their identification with it. They do not need the baby to give thanks to them, because they themselves feel the thanks. They are the baby as well as the comforting, nursing, protecting mother. They do not need any more communications from the baby than they need from their own arms and legs.

Some mothers, however, are quite frightened by the baby at this stage, primarily because they see in it an example of primitive instinctuality which is uncontrolled. If they have problems in regard to their capacity to control instinctual impulses, close contact with this situation is likely to stimulate deep fears. These usually show themselves in one of two ways. Either the mother reacts irrationally to the baby, as though the baby were a dangerous object who will do her some harm, and as though it were full of uncontrollable hostility; or else she feels the uncontrollable hostility inside herself, and she fears to go near the baby lest she take advantage of its helplessness, and harm it. In extreme cases there actually are mothers who do harm their babies; but these cases are rare. Much more common are those in which this mechanism is present to the extent that it obtrudes between mother and child, and prevents or delays the building up of a relationship between them until after this stage has passed, that is to say, until after the baby has ceased to be the little uncontrollable bundle. The doctors and the nurses who have known the mothers during pregnancy will probably already have been warned to expect such a situation, because the mothers will either have voiced explicit fears of small babies or they will have talked about fantasies of their babies-to-be in terms which have pointedly excluded infants of under three or four months. I mentioned this group in Chapter 3. They never fantasy a baby of under three or four months. When you find that during pregnancy, you watch out for trouble after birth.

The management of this type of situation should focus upon reassurance regarding the harmlessness of close contact between mother and child; but there is no point in pushing the child into the mother's arms faster than she can bear it, because, apart from the fact that it would not work anyway, and it would very likely make her more frightened, we know that these particular stimuli coming from the child, namely that the child is an uncontrollable bundle of instincts, will change within three or four months, and then the mother's pattern is likely to alter spontaneously. If the mother is allowed to, as it were, coast along until the baby is three or four months old, then this particular frightening stimulation from the baby will disappear, and the main source of the mother's fears will go at the same time.

Another source of difficulty during this first stage is caused by the infant's lack of capacity to communicate. This worries most mothers, as evidenced by the universal joy on the occasion of the infant's first smile. I am interested in the tremendous effect this has on mothers. We all know mothers who will say, 'My baby smiled at one week old', and someone else says, 'No, that was wind.' But why are they so interested in this smile? I think it is because they now feel the baby can show gratitude in a person-alized way. It is interesting that most mothers feel quite differ-ently about the smile from the way they feel about the sight of a baby who is flushed, peaceful, and gratified, after having been successfully fed. If you contrast this with the raging, howling, ravenous creature of half an hour ago and say, 'Here we can see what the effect of feeding is', this does not mean nearly as much to them as the smile of the child after he has been fed.

Although the majority of mothers are dissatisfied that their babies cannot talk to them in the early stages, they are able to put up with this frustration, or to defend themselves against it, by imaginary happy conversations with the baby. You all know how young mothers constantly talk to their babies; and people who are standing by listening think they are a bit silly. 'What is all this nonsense? She talks, and then she answers as though from the baby. The conversation is all coming from her. What is this play-acting?' This play-acting is the mother's attempt to over-come the frustration that she feels because the baby cannot talk to her. Some mothers, especially those who are young and inex-perienced, and have feelings of unworthiness or self-depreciation, cannot comfort themselves in this way. If they were to have imaginary conversations, their babies would be accusing them of not having done enough for them. They pass through agonies of doubt as to their capacities for motherhood. They suspect that their milk is too weak, or is insufficient in quantity. They are afraid of their clumsiness in handling the baby, and so on. Moreover, they feel that they are being called upon by the baby to give and give all the time, twenty-four hours a day, and seven days a week. And they see no return from the baby. The baby does not express thanks. They get no reassurance from the baby that they are doing the right thing. It is true that every now and again they get some assurance from the approving word of the nurse or the paediatrician, and if they weigh the baby they can watch its weight on the chart and see that it is increasing; but they are in need of more frequent immediate communication; and they are especially in need of emotional supplies which the baby will inject later on into the circular system, when it can communicate with them.

As we talk about this group of mothers, it becomes clear that we are talking about a continuation of that passivity and introversion that we saw during pregnancy. And again, just as in pregnancy, it is necessary to gratify this. With these mothers after the birth of the baby it is often necessary to gratify these dependent wishes. Physicians and nurses can be especially helpful, during this preliminary stage of motherhood, by continual and unstinting support. The mothers can also be helped educationally by assisting them to learn the behavioural cues of the baby which can be used instead of communication to determine that all is progressing well. A good deal of the education in a well-baby clinic has this particular goal. The mother should herself be able to recognize that all is going well; and she should not have to wait for the end of the week to come and see the nurse and the paediatrician, so that they should tell her that everything is in order. It is also useful if the caretaking agents can mobilize the sources of love and affection for the mother in her circle of family and friends, and particularly in her relationship with her husband.

Paediatricians are sometimes worried by the burden of satisfying the apparently insatiable dependent needs of such mothers at this time. They may feel that the mother should be able to stand on her own feet as soon as possible; and with the constant demands of a busy practice, it is hard to be constantly on the phone answering the apparently childish questions of an over-anxious young mother. But I think that many experienced paediatricians realize that satisfying the mother's needs at this time of crisis will have a far-reaching effect in increasing her self-esteem, so that when the baby does begin to communicate with her, she will already have gained the confidence in her own worth which will promote a positive basis for the developing relationship. This resembles the case of a baby with a constitutionally intense need to suck. If this need to suck is gratified at the beginning of life, the child will not be a thumb-sucker afterwards, whereas if it is not gratified, he will usually suck his thumb for a long time.

From three Months to seven Months

We now come to the smoothest and happiest phase, namely from about three to seven months. This is the phase of the 'perfect baby'. He begins to develop an obvious personality, and he shows signs of recognition and love for his mother. He is usually adapted to extra-uterine life by now, and he is adapted to the feeding situation. His development is exciting and rapid and very obvious, and yet it does not involve him in creating a nuisance. He lies happily in his crib most of his waking hours fascinated by his play with simple things, by his fingers and toes and the sights around him. He begins to babble and vocalize and play with sounds in a way that delights the heart of any mother. In fact he fits easily into most mothers' stereotype of the ideal trouble-free baby. Although he is still dependent upon his mother, she sees that he is rapidly developing control over his functions, and his demands on her are not continuous and insistent, so that she can sometimes get a rest from her mothering duties.

The only area where difficulties are at all common during this period is in the baby's sleeping habits. Mothers may need paediatric help in regulating the baby's rhythm so that he sleeps at night and is awake during the day. This process may be occasionally interfered with in quite a characteristic way by sexual problems between the parents. Worry about the wakefulness of the baby may be used vicariously by the mother to avoid working through difficulties with her husband which would otherwise emerge at night. It is not at all unusual to find the baby's wakefulness being used as a contra-coital defence, and mothers will tell you that the baby cries all night and this is a great shame because her husband has to work in the day; and so she has to put the husband in another room far away where he can sleep undisturbed. This mother will tell you that the baby wakes every hour on the hour; and so she has to wake up herself every hour in order to make sure whether the baby is asleep. As she talks to you, you discover that sometimes when she wakes up, the baby is not actually awake, but he is lying a bit crooked in his bed, and so she has to straighten him, or put the blanket back on, and that wakes him up.

This situation is a sample of the main difficulties which occur during this period. The mother may have no serious complaints about the child, quite the contrary. But since his needs are at this time not obtrusive, there is the possibility that he may be woven more easily into a vicarious solution of some non-maternal problems of his mother. The result of this process in distorting the mother-child relationship may not be obvious until later. On the whole, however, this period is one which is conducive to laying down a confident relaxed type of reciprocal relationship, in which neither party makes any undue demands, and in which both can express their gratification and produce a benign reverberation.

The only real danger of this phase is associated with this very gratification. If the mother, for some personality reason, or because of emotional deprivation in other current relationships, cannot handle the frustration of the next stage, she may become fixated at this second phase; and either try to prevent the child moving out of the 'perfect baby' stage, or else react with excessive disappointment and rejection when he starts growing away from her towards the end of the first year. The very experience of extra gratification in this phase may make it harder for her to step into the cold water, as it were, of the next stage.

From seven Months to twelve Months

The growing away of the child from the mother is the main characteristic of the third phase of the first year. The pleasant sucking of the middle phase turns to biting, and this is accompanied by many other signs that the baby is developing a will of his own which may not be entirely in line with his mother's wishes. His capacity for aggressive expression begins to develop. Teeth appear, neuro-muscular development allows him to stand on his own, and towards the end of the year he takes his first steps. These are greeted by most mothers with delight; but they soon realize that these are the first steps that the baby is taking away from them. Similarly, the baby's control over urination is a sign of growing independence, but this usually leads on to the inevitable conflicts of bladder-training. The mother is overjoyed when the baby develops the capacity for verbal communication; but the word 'no' appears fairly early in the second year.

The third phase of the first year is therefore a period of transition between the dependent trouble-free infant, and the toddler who is still dependent, but showing already the signs of future independence. This is the stage when the stimuli from the child increase the pressure toward the diatrophic and away from the symbiotic type of relationship and when the mother first faces the necessity of striking an appropriate balance between control and gratification of the child's impulses, as well as satisfaction of his dependence and provision of freedom for independent expression, which are essential parts of the task of parenthood. At this stage, too, the child begins to build up relationships with others besides his mother, and if she has not in the past been able to come to terms with rivalry situations, she may have difficulty in accepting this. The good-humoured arguments as to whether the baby learns to say 'mama' before 'dada' may symbolize deeper jealousies. This is a time when maternal over-possessiveness may first be seen and, if recognized, may be most appropriately dealt with by the educational efforts of paediatricians and nurses.

I will interrupt my description of the developing mother-child relationship at this point because I wish to take up another topic which is allied to it, namely, the effects of mother-child separation.

MOTHER-CHILD SEPARATION

In talking about the effects of mother-child separation, I should like to refer to John Bowlby's *Maternal Care and Mental Health* (1951), which I have for many years felt to be probably the most important and fundamental textbook in the mental health field. I shall begin my short discussion of this topic with an extract from that book because it summarizes the situation quite succinctly, and, as usual with Bowlby, in beautiful language.

> 'What is believed to be essential to mental health is that the infant and young child should experience a warm, intimate, and continuous relationship with his mother (or permanent mother-substitute) in which both find satisfaction and enjoyment. Given this relationship, the emotions of anxiety and guilt, which in excess characterize mental ill-health, will develop in a moderate and organized way. When this happens, the child's characteristic and contradictory demands, on the one hand for unlimited love from his parents and on the other for revenge upon them when he feels that they do not love him enough, will likewise remain of moderate strength and become amenable to the control of his gradually developing personality' (Bowlby, 1951, p. 11).

That is to me a beautiful sentence, because in it Bowlby summarizes a major contribution of the psycho-analytic school of psychology to our understanding of the earlier stages of infant personality development. These contradictory demands on the one hand for unlimited love, and on the other hand for revenge because no baby does get unlimited love, lead to inevitable conflicts at the beginning of life. How these conflicts are resolved will determine to a large extent what happens in regard to future personality development. It may be recalled that, in the discussion in Chapter 2 about reactions to the loss of a loved person, I said that one of the important factors which determines the outcome was how this particular set of conflicts was handled right at the beginning of life. How it was handled at the beginning of life will depend to a considerable extent on the interchange which took place in the reality of the child-rearing process between the infant and its mother. It is this complex relationship with the mother in the early years, varied in countless ways by relations with the father and the siblings, that child psychiatrists now believe to mould the development of the core of the personality.

Bowlby goes on to say:

'A state of affairs in which the child does not have this relationship is termed "maternal deprivation". This is a general term covering a number of different situations. Thus, a child is deprived even though living at home if his mother (or permanent mother-substitute) is unable to give him the loving care small children need. Again, a child is deprived if for any reason he is removed from his mother's care. This deprivation will be relatively mild if he is then looked after by someone whom he has already learned to know and trust, but may be considerable if the foster-mother, even though loving, is a stranger. All these arrangements, however, give the child some satisfaction and are therefore examples of partial deprivation. They stand in contrast to the almost complete deprivation which is still not uncommon in institutions, residential nurseries, and hospitals, where the child often has no one who cares for him in a personal way and with whom he may feel secure.

'The ill-effects of deprivation vary with its degree. Partial deprivation brings in its train acute anxiety, excessive need for love, powerful feelings of revenge, and, arising from these last, guilt and depression. These emotions and drives are too great for the immature means of control and organization available to the young child. The consequent disturbance of psychic organization then leads to a variety of responses, often repetitive and cumulative, the end products of which are symptoms of neurosis and instability of character. Complete deprivation, with which we shall be dealing principally in this report, has even more far-reaching effects on character development and may entirely cripple the capacity to make relationships' (Bowlby, 1951, pp. 11–12).

Bowlby then goes on to discuss the classes of evidence which are available from all parts of the world in regard to the noxious pathogenic effects of prolonged mother-child separation.

'Evidence that the deprivation of mother-love in early childhood can have a far-reaching effect on the mental health and personality development of human beings comes from many sources. It falls into three main classes: [Firstly] . . . studies, by direct observation, of the mental health and development of children in institutions, hospitals, and foster-homes. [These are called *direct studies*. Secondly] . . . studies which investigate the early histories of adolescents or adults who have developed psychological illnesses [*retrospective studies*]' (Bowlby, 1951, p. 15).

One example of this second kind of study is Bowlby's first work, written up in a book called *Forty-four Juvenile Thieves* (Bowlby, 1946). Working in a child guidance clinic, he discovered that there was a group of delinquent children who resembled each other in certain characteristics, mainly in regard to the fact that they were what he called 'affectionless', they were unable to feel affection for anyone. When he investigated the past histories of these children, he discovered that there was one common characteristic in a statistically significant proportion of them, namely, that they had been separated from their mothers, or mother-figures, for periods of more than three or four months before the age of five years. The third class of studies is composed of those studies which *follow up* groups of children who have suffered deprivation in early years, with a view to determining their state of mental health.

'The direct studies are the most numerous. They make it plain that, when deprived of maternal care, the child's development is almost always retarded – physically, intellectually, and socially – and that symptoms of physical and mental illness may appear. Such evidence is disquieting, but sceptics may question whether the retardation is permanent and whether the symptoms of illness may not easily be overcome. The retrospective and follow-up studies make it clear that such optimism is not always justified and that some children are gravely damaged for life. This is a sombre conclusion which must now be regarded as established.

'There are, however, important features of the situation about which little is known. For instance, it is by no means clear why some children succumb and some do not. It may be that hereditary factors play a part, but, before resorting to a principle which has been so readily invoked as a universal solvent of biological problems, it is important to review what is known of the effects of such factors as the child's age, and the length and, especially, the degree, of his deprivation, each of which there is reason to think is vital' (Bowlby, 1951, pp. 15–16).

I do not wish to go 'through a discussion of all these studies, which are probably familiar to you. I may say that the conclusion Bowlby stated so emphatically in 1951 when he wrote this has been questioned by other people in recent years; and in recent months, other workers have thrown some doubt on the certainty with which one can say that mother-child separation is an inevitable pathogenic factor. I think that many of these doubts are based on the fact that people are using one of the old theoretical models of stress. The assumption is that when certain individuals are faced by stress this is pathogenic. Therefore, you would expect that a high proportion of them, or a significant proportion of them, according to how great the stress is, will be damaged. That is the simple model. It is a bit different from the model which I discussed in Chapter 2, which is the model of crisis. When stress is regarded as a precipitant of a crisis, we realize that the outcome may in certain cases be pathological, but there is also the possibility that the crisis may be weathered in a positive manner. This is a different type of model. In one model you expect that you do some damaging thing to people, and maybe someone escapes, but you expect the majority of them to suffer as a result. In the other model you present people with hazard, and then they go into a crisis situation. Then, dependent upon what happens during the crisis, which is itself dependent upon many factors which we have already discussed, a certain proportion will come out damaged, some will come out unchanged, and a certain proportion will come out improved. My feeling is that some of the recent work, which attempts to reduce our estimation of the importance of mother-child separation, is based upon the earlier model. Some workers feel that if you can show that out of a hundred children exposed to mother-child separation not all are damaged, but only perhaps thirty per cent, you can say that this is not a very important matter. And especially if you can show that some of these children were not only not damaged, but even improved as a result of this process, you may say, 'Well mother-child separation is of very little consequence.'

'A Two-year-old Goes to Hospital'

Be that as it may, I should like to discuss briefly one of the most interesting types of study in this field, namely, one of the current studies to observe what happens when a child is separated from its mother. This has been studied extensively at the Tavistock Clinic in London by Bowlby and his colleagues, and has been made the subject of two films by James Robertson. I am going to discuss one of these films, *A Two-year-old Goes to Hospital* (Robertson, 1953a).

It is quite an interesting film, incidentally, because it represents the lucky break of an amateur. Robertson was a social worker at the Tavistock Clinic concerned with research; and he got the notion that it might be a good idea to take a movie of a child who was separated from its mother. He had never done any photography, but he bought himself a camera, and he set up a situation to try out his camera and see whether he could get a film. *A Two-year-old Goes to Hospital* represents his first attempt. This was a practice attempt and the practice turned out so well that it was made into a permanent film. I have not seen his second film *Going to Hospital with Mother* (1958a), which he has made since he became a 'professional', photographer. I hope that it is as good as the first one.

The first film is a documentary account of what happens to a two-year five-month-old girl, a normal, bright, intelligent, nice-looking little girl, who was put into a hospital for seven days for a minor operation, which every paediatrician in the United States to whom I have spoken regards as unnecessary, and would never have been performed there. It was an operation for the repair of an umbilical hernia. This was a minor operation. It did not cause her much suffering. So the film is a documentary account mainly of separation of child from mother, and is complicated as little as possible by the child's suffering as the result of surgical interference.

This film illustrates three successive overlapping stages in the reaction of the child to the separation experience. First, there was the stage of *protest,* secondly, there was the stage of *despair,* and thirdly, there was the stage of *adaptation.*

The protest period started at the moment the child realized she was being separated from her mother; and as those of you who saw the film will remember, she came to the hospital all right, and she went along with the nurse without trouble. Her mother stayed behind, and she was taken by the nurse into a room where she was given a bath, and that was where she started crying violently and saying repeatedly, 'I want my mummy.' She went on crying and screaming this way, with periods of quiescence, for about two to four days. The real period of protest in this child was about two days, but there were hints of it for the next day or two. There is evidence from other sources that this protest is stronger the closer the bond between mother and child, and the less the child has in the past been separated from his mother.

The next stage is the stage of despair. Following the stage of protest, the child becomes depressed and resigned; and in the film you will remember that this was especially well shown because this little child had very expressive features. As you watched her facial expressions, and even her bodily stance, you could see her, as the days went on, sagging lower and lower, and her face showed more and more depression. During this period there are signs of hostility, which the child directs towards the mother, or the mother-substitute, or towards herself; and it is this hostility which is the main cause, we think, of the depression. The child harbours fantasies such as 'I'm a bad girl, and that is why my mummy has thrown me out.' You will recall in the film the way in which the child was attempting to conquer the feeling of depression. You saw her trying to smile, and trying to play. Sometimes she jumped up and down, and made gestures as though she were happy, and as she was doing this she suddenly drooped and she really looked very sad indeed.

This was a very well-behaved little girl, she did not show too much aggression, but she showed it when they gave her the doll, the big doll they used for practising nursing procedures. They gave her this beautiful big doll to play with, and she started beating the doll up. On another occasion, her mother came and brought her a picture book, and as soon as her mother left she started tearing this up. The other way in which she showed her hostility towards her mother was that she kept saying, 'I want my mummy, I want my mummy', but when her mother came, she turned her head away. She showed much less hostility to the father when he came. This was interesting. She blamed the mother for leaving her, but when father came she immediately had a relationship with him. When mother visited she would turn away, and it took the mother some hard work for a few minutes before she could persuade her to relate to her.

Then we come to the third stage, the phase of adaptation. The phase of adaptation may occur within about a week from the onset of separation, and it is characterized by a denial of affection for the mother, and a denial of the need for the mother, and of the need for a relationship with a mother-person. When this state continues for a long time it produces a distortion of personality development. The child is blocking off one of the main avenues of personality growth, he is pushing the mother out; and is, by pushing the mother out, pushing away everyone, except in quite a superficial paper-thin type of relationship. The child dissociates bodily and sensual stimulation from the building-up and maintenance of a relationship with another person. He becomes self-sufficient, and this eventually leads to affectionless traits of character, which have been described by so many workers as the main characteristic of the pathological sequelae of prolonged separation from the mother in early childhood. In the film the child's turning away from the mother when she first came in for her visits was the first sign of this denial of the mother. It was a sign of hostility towards the mother that was also an adaptation; because one way the child can overcome her depression is to feel, 'I'm not miserable because mummy isn't here, because I don't need her. In fact I don't need anyone, I'm all right by myself, and I don't need others', which we see very well developed in certain delinquent personalities, whose delinquency is based upon the fact that they do not internalize the values of society. This kind of personality distortion is an exaggerated end-result of what we saw in its early stages in this normal little girl who was separated for only seven days from her mother.

If the separation experience is not too prolonged, the child apparently reverts to his previous psychological functioning within a week or two after he returns home to his mother. During the initial back home period, the child is usually negativistic, and 'fails to recognize his mother'. This is one of the most painful things for mothers. He recognizes other people, and of course he really recognizes his mother, but he pretends he does not. Following that, when he begins to recognize his mother, he becomes overly dependent, and he grabs hold of her skirts and will not let her out of his sight. When she wants to go to the bathroom, he kicks up a fuss because he wants to go with her wherever she goes. This behaviour is a source of considerable strain for some mothers, they just do not know what has come over their child, why he is grabbing at them the whole time.

The length of the separation time needed to produce protracted or irreversible psychological manifestations varies with the age of the child. The younger the child, the less separation time needed to produce pathology. Most children under three suffer permanently some personality defects from separation of several weeks or more. When I say *most* children it is based upon the earlier studies. I think some of the later studies would throw doubt on that; but if it is not most children who suffer ill effects it is a significant proportion. The majority of children between three and five sustain some damage; and it is probable that only a minority between five and eight emerge with defects. These proportions still await confirmation; and we really need some more research to find out what the epidemiological story is in these cases. All we can say is that, under three, the probability of continuing damage is greater; from three to five there is possibility of damage; and from five on there is much less possibility, unless there is quite prolonged separation.

DISCUSSION

Question: Dr. Caplan, I have a real question, and this has to do with when should a mother go back to work after the birth of her baby?

Answer: Well, I cannot answer the question as put, 'When should the mother go back to work?', because this is a question which has clearly economic and social and psychological factors involved in it, and cultural factors too. All I can do is hazard a guess as to some of the psychological factors that have to be taken into account. One of them relates to the length of the work day, namely, how much is the mother going to be away from her baby? And the other relates to who can take care of the baby while she is away. Is the baby going to be taken care of in its own home, or removed and taken care of somewhere else? I think that what I could say in general without giving a whole lecture about this is, first, that during the first three to five months it is essential that the mother should stay at home, assuming she is going to be the mothering person. In other words, if the grandmother is the mothering person in the beginning, then it does not matter if the mother goes out to work at the end of the first week, but if the mother is the mothering person, then there should be a stable continuing relationship with the baby during that first period of three to five months. This is the essential period when the baby is building up the core of its personality, and it should be relating to one person. Some years ago we would not have said this. We were very much impressed by the fact that a baby at this stage does not relate to a whole object, to a whole mother. It relates to the smell separately, and the sight separately, and the feel separately, and the temperature separately. So people said that as long as the baby got all the stimulation that it needed, and all the food that it needed, and all the comfort that it needed, it did not make any difference whether you changed it around from one person to another. We now realize that this is quite wrong, that this is indeed a very sensitive period when we want to help the baby to unite the separate sensory impressions into one whole person; because the integrity of the baby's personality depends on his being able to weld these sensations together into one whole object. So during this period it is very important that the same mothering person should continue all the way through. When you get beyond that stage, our experience shows that the mother can go away for certain periods during the day, as long as there is a stable substitute who will give personalized care. The child will then relate both to the primary mothering person and to a secondary mothering person. In those circumstances, the mother can go out to work at that stage as far as psychological factors are concerned, as long as she is able to maintain continuing relations with her child during part of the day. His own home is best, a foster-home is slightly less good; but a foster-home is much better than placing him in a nursery. Placing him in a nursery during the day is much better than putting him in a residential nursery, where his mother will see him only at the weekends, or once or twice during the week. There are all gradations here, and what I am giving you are my hunches. There is relatively little evidence from scientific studies as yet to support this view. There are, however, some studies, particularly by Heinicke (1956) at the Tavistock Clinic, showing that there is a difference in the reaction of children in residential nurseries as compared with children in day nurseries. The children in residential nurseries show, at quite an early age, a less satisfactory development than the others. And the others show less satisfactory development than a control group of healthy children in their own homes. Nevertheless, I would inject one other note of caution. No one can be very dogmatic in this area, because it depends very much on the general cultural situation. I have carried out studies in the communal settlements in Israel, where children from birth are brought up in institutions, but where their parents have access to them frequently during the day; and there is no doubt that these particular children in their early years seem to show some signs of deprivation, but they get over this quite well, because of the unique living situation in the settlements.

Question: What is the influence of a broken home?

Answer: By a broken home, you mean a home where there is no father? I hope to discuss this later [Chapter 5] when we talk about the integrity of the family, but briefly I would say in regard to the present topic that absence of a father weakens the mother very considerably during this first year of life, because she does not have the active support of the man in the home. However, it means much more later on in the child's life because the father role is an active role in the bringing up of the child. He is not important to the child directly in the first year. He is of secondary importance through his support of his wife, and his satisfaction of her dependency needs, so that she can then satisfy the child's dependency needs. But later on in the child's life, the father role, as a separate role, is important. If he is missing, the mother has to play both the mother role and also the father role, which is a great strain on her. She cannot do it completely. She cannot act as a model of masculinity, either for her son to copy or for her daughter to learn what maleness is.

Question: Children in hospital cry after visiting hours. Is this a valid reason for restricting visits?

Answer: I think this is a very good question. Parting is painful both for the child and the mother. Should we, because of this, restrict visiting in order not to hurt them? I think the tone of the question presupposes that pain is a natural psychobiological response, and it is a very useful response. Pain tells us that we have a painful situation to which we must adapt and adjust. We must realize that two people who can part without pain have no relationship. 'Parting is such sweet sorrow . . .', and the very deep implication of this is that the parting is not only sorrow; and it is sweet because it implies a relationship. Avoiding pain in this situation is like avoiding causing pain to a young mother who has just given birth to a deformed child, by keeping the child away from her. Well, we do avoid giving her pain in that way, but we also avoid stimulating her to adjust to the painful reality. So the argument that we must restrict visiting because it is painful is the same argument as people give in the lying-in hospital, 'You must not allow the mother to see her deformed child because that is painful.' That kind of pain in a child after visiting, although unpleasant, is the kind of pain that I, as a psychiatrist, like to see. I am not sadistic, but I like to see that pain because when I see it I know that the child continues its relationship with the mother, and the mother continues her relationship with the child; and that they are being forced by this stimulation to adjust to the unpleasant realities of life, namely, that they are separated. And when I do not see the pain, I, as a psychiatrist, get worried lest the relationship has been interrupted; and if it has been interrupted in the child, I get worried that the child's relationships with everyone else will also be interrupted.

Question: Is it a good idea for the mother to be in and out of the ward the whole time, or should visiting hours be restricted?

Answer: This depends on cultural and social and economic factors. As a psychiatrist, I would much rather see the kind of institution where the mother is actively involved in the nursing of her child, which is happening in certain modern paediatric hospitals, and where the separation is cut down to the lowest possible amount within the reality of the situation. Now this, of course, implies a tremendous change from our traditions in the way in which such an institution is administered. In some paediatric hospitals facilities have been arranged for the mothers to take an active part during the twenty-four hours in the care of their children, and all the reports that I have seen indicate that although this requires considerable readjustment of the culture of the institution there have been nothing but happy results.

REFERENCES

BOWLBY, JOHN (1946). *Forty-four Juvenile Thieves*. London: Baillière, Tindall & Cox.

BOWLBY, JOHN (1951). *Maternal Care and Mental Health*. Geneva: World Health Organization; London: H.M.S.O.; New York: Columbia University Press. Abridged Version, *Child Care and the Growth of Love*. Harmondsworth: Pelican Books A 271, 1953.

CAPLAN, GERALD (1959). *Concepts of Mental Health and Consultation*. Washington, D.C.: Children's Bureau Publication No. 373.

HEINICKE, C. M. (1956). 'Some Effects of Separating Two-year-old Children from their Parents: a Comparative Study.' *Hum. Relat.* **9**, 105.

ROBERTSON, JAMES (1953a). Film: *A Two-year-old Goes to Hospital*. 16mm. Snd. 45 mins. English or French. London: Tavistock Clinic; New York University Film Library.

ROBERTSON, JAMES (1953b). Guide to the film *A Two-year-old Goes to Hospital*. London: Tavistock Publications.

ROBERTSON, JAMES (1958a). Film: *Going to Hospital with Mother*. 16mm. Snd. 45 mins. London: Tavistock Institute of Human Relations; New York University Film Library.

ROBERTSON, JAMES (1958b). *Young Children in Hospital*. London: Tavistock Publications; New York: Basic Books, under the title *Young Children in Hospitals*.

CHAPTER 5

Mental Health Aspects of Family Life

In this chapter I wish to pull together some of the loose threads of the previous discussions in regard to emotional interrelations in the family and their effect on the mental health of the children and the other members. One of the simple insights about the mental health implications of family life which we have developed in recent years is that you should not just focus on one particular referent person such as a child in whom you are interested, and operate as though the rest of the family has meaning only in relation to him. Even if you do that, you will eventually come round to examining the mental health of every single member of the family, and you will find yourself also studying the mental health of the family as a group, as a small unit of society with a culture of its own.

It is much easier if you start off with the latter point of view, by widening your focus to include every member in the family, and by realizing that everyone in the family has psychological needs that have to be satisfied. The family group is an interdependent system. What affects any one member affects everyone.

So far we have concentrated on the mother-child relationship, and have spelled out the importance for mental health of what goes on between these two people. We have also emphasized that their relationship is influenced by the mother's relationship with her husband, and with her other children, and by their relationships with each other. Any two-person relationship in the family is affected by all the other two-person relationships.

In addition, the whole group has a unity of its own. It has

certain traditions and values, a unique history, special ways of running its life, certain ways of communicating among its members, and idiosyncratic leadership patterns. It is clear that we are talking about a whole system, not about mother and father only, or mother and child, or father and child. There are things that go on in this group, as there are that go on in all groups, which can be analysed in terms of the transactions of the group, rather than in terms of what any particular person does. It is similar to talking about the social system of a community in comparing, let us say, Denver with Central City, or Denver with Los Angeles. Each of these cities has a characteristic way of life, a characteristic culture, and characteristic traditions which influence all the people who live there. This way of life is, of course, itself influenced by these people, but not just by the people living there at present. The way of life in Denver is determined also by the people who lived in Denver in the past who laid out the city in a special way, and built buildings of a certain shape, and designed parks in a characteristic way, and excluded industry up to a certain time, and so on. So the history of the city has had an effect on the present-day inhabitants, in the same way that the history of a family, including all the influences, biological, psychological, economic, and social, which have impinged upon it in the past, will affect its present way of life; and its present way of life will affect the details of what goes on nowadays in regard to any particular individual in that family.

We tend sometimes to talk about a family as though it were a static entity. But of course everyone knows that a family has a life history of its own as a unit. It has a beginning, a middle, and an end. Some people have studied this by dividing the whole family system into sub-systems. They say the family has a marital system, a parent-child system, and a sibling system, and they trace the separate development over time of each of these sub-systems, and their influence upon each other. They point out that at the beginning of the emergence of a family, the marital system, the relation of the man and the woman who become the husband and the wife, is a close system. The wife emerges from her family of origin, the husband leaves his family; and they are

134

enabled to do this because of the close link they make with each other.

In the second phase of the history of a family the marital system becomes distant. As the parent-child system appears in the family, the marital system loosens, and this facilitates a close relationship between each of the parents and the children. This is the middle phase of family life.

Eventually the children leave the family, through marriage or through growing up and leaving home, and then the marital system closes up again.

Now, as in most aspects of development, previous phases influence subsequent phases. If there is a disorder, or a lack of satisfactory resolution of problems in a previous phase, it will affect subsequent phases; so that, for example, if the marital system was not initially close enough difficulties will appear in the subsequent family life. Now what might lead to the marital system not being close enough? This might happen if one of the marital partners retains too close a relationship with his previous system; if the mother, for example, does not emerge adequately from her family, or if some representative of this previous family intrudes into the present system and keeps the marital system from becoming close. We are very familiar with the pattern of the mother's mother, or the father's mother, living nearby and coming into the system. She then may keep the marital pair apart at the beginning when they should be close together. This leads to a disturbance of the trajectory of family life because the husband or wife has not managed to emancipate himself or herself either physically, or psychologically, or culturally, or economically from his or her own family.

Just to make the picture a little more complicated, when the man and the woman come into their new marital system, they may bring with them problems which were unresolved in the previous families; and these may exert a disturbing influence. I think it is very important to emphasize that this difficulty is not inevitable. If a woman comes from a disturbed family, or if a man comes from a disturbed family, there is an increased likelihood that their marital system may be interfered with. But there is equally the possibility that their pre-existing disturbance will be put right in this new system. We cannot predict, on the basis of knowing that a man and woman come from families in both of which there may have been difficulties, that they are necessarily going to have difficulties in their new marital system. The latter is a new entity, and there is the possibility, which I have emphasized through all the preceding chapters, that in this new situation better solutions will be found for the old problems than in the past. That explains why it is not infrequent to find a girl who was quite a disturbed person as a result of difficulties in her parents' home, marrying a man of the appropriate kind and making a new life with him, with the result that she matures. If you see her in three or four years' time, especially after the parent-child system has come into operation, and she has had an opportunity to work through some later phases, you may find that she has spontaneously matured, and the new marital system may not at all repeat the difficulties of the marital system of her parents. This is a good thing, because otherwise family life would gradually go downhill. If it were not for this, each generation would inherit the defects of the previous one, and gradually get more and more disorganized. But we must realize that each new family has the possibility of controlling its own fate to a considerable extent.

When the parent-child system comes into operation in the middle phase of the life of a family, if the marital system does not open up sufficiently, we are likely to find difficulties. We sometimes find that a husband and wife are so very closely attached to each other that the advent of children is regarded by them as an interference. They are interested in satisfying each other's needs completely, and children are in the way. In ordinary circumstances, when the children arrive, these people change their role from being husband and wife to becoming father and mother. As such they have more, as it were, within their emotional purview than when they were husband and wife. They play their part in two systems in the family, and they now share their psychological energies, which previously were concentrated on each other, between each other and the children.

Let us now discuss the third phase. When the children leave home, if the marital system does not close up, we find one of the results which we talked about previously. First of all the children are delayed from leaving home because the parent-child system keeps hold of them; and secondly, after the children leave home the parents follow the children out. Unless the parents at this stage can find each other again, and refocus their affectional ties on each other, they are apt to extend beyond the boundaries of their system, and interfere with the new systems that are forming as a result of their children leaving home, which gets us back to where we started.

I have forgotten who it was who thought out this way of looking at the family, I think it was Norman Polansky, and I feel that it is quite a good way of talking about the recurring patterns in the natural histories of families.

I have talked a good deal in this and earlier chapters about the psychological needs of people. I have stressed the thesis that mental health is dependent upon the satisfactory gratification of certain fundamental needs.

You will remember that Bowlby also talked about this in that excerpt quoted from his book in Chapter 4. What are these psychological needs? Clearly people have physical needs too, and unless these are satisfied they are apt to deteriorate in one way or another, and this has also to be borne in mind, but for the moment, I am going to concentrate on the psychological needs. We can say that there are certain requisites in the social milieu of a person, and if these requisites are not present difficulties arise. One of the most fundamental prerequisites for health is that there should in fact be a social milieu. We have come to realize that a person cannot exist in a state of mental health without interaction with other people. We psychiatrists have come to recognize this quite recently as a result of experiments that were carried out originally in Canada, and later in Bethesda, and since then in many different places.

In these experiments volunteers were isolated for varying lengths of time from physical stimulation and from interaction with other people. In the Canadian experiment medical students

137

were shut up in soundproof rooms with their eyes and ears covered. They were kept in these rooms for two or three days, and no one talked to them. They were just handed their food at intervals, and that was the only contact they had with the outside world. It was discovered that these medical students fairly rapidly became extremely uncomfortable and quite disturbed psychologically. It varied from one student to the next, but usually after one to three days the students began to manifest psychosis-like symptoms. They became disorientated, they became confused, and they began to hallucinate.

The people in Bethesda went one better, they did not use volunteers, they did it themselves. One psychiatrist suspended himself in a big tank of warm water. His only contact with his surroundings was through a rubber tube which fed him air. It was all dark and soundproof. He was just floating around in the middle of this warm water. He discovered that he began to have psychotic symptoms within about two hours and he began to have hallucinations.

From experiments such as these we are discovering that we need a constant level of sensory input in order to keep our psychological machine going in the ordinary way. If you cut sensory stimulation down you run into gross disturbance in the psychological sphere. If you allow sensory stimulation but do not have social stimulation, you also run into difficulty. So the first priority of need is for adequate sensory stimulation, and the second priority is for stimulation by other people.

I was at a meeting of the Group for the Advancement of Psychiatry where Dr. Lilley from Bethesda was talking about this research, and I came home very excited because, from the psychiatric point of view, this was very important work indeed. My daughter, who was then about thirteen, said to me, 'Daddy, where have you been?' and I told her. And she said, 'What was it all about?' and I described to her the isolation experiments and their results, and she said, 'You psychiatrists, you're always finding out things that everyone knows!' So I asked her what she meant. 'Well,' she answered, 'everyone knows that isolation produces mental disorder. Look at Treasure Island, look at Ben

Gunn, he was marooned on the island, and didn't he go crazy; and look at all the prisoners they put in dungeons, and don't they go crazy?' And she was quite right. Of course we have always known this. It was just that the psychiatrists did not know it!

So we have carried out a lot of complicated scientific experiments, and we have discovered in scientific words what the people have known for as long as history, namely, that isolation is a punishing and a traumatic phenomenon. But when we begin to examine it a little more closely, I feel, despite what my daughter said, that it was important that these experiments were carried out; because we are now beginning to tease these processes apart, and to find out exactly why it is that isolation is traumatic, and what are the pathways whereby isolation leads to these particular pathological manifestations.

As we begin to tease them apart, we discover that there is a whole complicated set of operations that goes on between two people, and if it does not go on we run into psychological difficulties. From this work we begin to realize the importance of operations which previously went on silently so that we did not notice them. In the same way, until the work of Bowlby and Spitz and others, no one really paid any scientific attention to the importance of the mother-child relationship.

So it is possible to make a list of the interpersonal requisites which are necessary for the satisfactory mental equilibrium of people. Many workers have made such lists, and they are shorter or longer, according to the different way they cut the cake. I have my own list. I just give it to you for what it is worth. Take into account that I am perfectly willing to make my categories bigger or smaller. I list seven requisites, but I am prepared to cut the cake differently in order to have twelve or twenty.

Love. First, there is the need for *love*, whatever that is. I find it hard to define, but I hope that everyone reading this book has from his own experience some idea of what I am talking about. I would here point out one other thing, and that is that these needs are needs which children have, but they are just as much needs that adults have. Not only children but adults too need love. Sometimes we tend to forget that adults have psychological needs. The category of love includes the need to be loved, and also the need to love. There is a recipient and a giving side in loving, and if either aspect is disturbed difficulties will result.

Support forms the second category. Love, in so far as one can define it, means love for one's own sake irrespective of what one does. Support, on the other hand, is in direct relationship to what you do. You need to be supported in regard to a task, or to support someone else in regard to a task. Another way of talking about support is as a need to be dependent upon someone else. But one also has a need for independence. One has a need to be able to accomplish a task on one's own, to stand on one's own two feet. Here we come into a rather complicated area. The ratio of needs for dependence and independence varies among different people at different stages of their life. According to the degree of ego strength (see Chapter 2) and according to the degree of maturation, there has to be a different equilibrium between the need to be dependent and the need to be independent; so that adults need less support and more opportunity to be independent than children. But anyone who thinks that you ever become entirely independent is making a big mistake. Adults, too, have dependency needs, have needs to be supported by others. They also have a need to support others; and very rapidly, even in childhood, children have the need to support others. They want to have younger children that they can help out.

Impulse control. Another pair of needs are also coupled in this same way. I talked in Chapter 2 about instinctual impulses, about various appetites and drives which have a rather primitive biological origin, sex drives, aggression, various bodily appetites for food, for stimulation of various sorts, and so on. Each person has a need to have these instinctual demands gratified, and he searches for gratification. But in addition, in our culture and in all societies, there is the need on the part of the individual to control these instinctual needs, demands, and impulses. This control is internalized; that is to say, the person controls himself, and this is one aspect of ego functioning. But interestingly enough, there is also the need to have outside help with the control of these impulses, help from other people, and help from the customs and traditions of society. Since it seems a reasonable theory that a good deal of the psychological energy which we use for socially accepted goals in our daily life comes originally from these primitive instinctual sources, it becomes clear that unless the instinctual impulses are controlled, and their strength drained off for useful purposes, we will not have the psychological energy for our everyday living.

The need to feel part of a group is a rather complicated one; not just to have a relationship with one person, or not just to have love; not just to be controlled, not just to have the possibility of gratifying instinctual demands, but a need of a higher order. This is the need to be part of a group, where one can feel free to relax, and where one can feel secure, where one can be buttressed by the presence of other people whom one trusts and, most important possibly, where one can get continual reassurance in regard to one's identity. This last point has been alluded to by Nathan Ackerman in his book *The Psychodynamics of Family Life* (1958). I will come back to what he says later. But I just want to spell out what is involved here. I have said that one of the special functions of the ego is the integration, the synthesis, of all that goes on in the person's life, of the external demands and pressures, and of the internal impulses, in order to produce some consistent pattern of functioning which gives an idiosyncratic pattern to the behaviour of that person, which we call his identity. And I have said that part of the ego's function is awareness of one's own identity, and confidence in one's identity. If this confidence is interfered with, then there is a weakening of the ego capacity to synthesize and to integrate all these manifold needs, and to produce an equilibrium as a resultant of all these complicated forces.

It would appear that most people need constant evidence from the outside world about their identity. If they are left entirely on their own, the capacity to be confident in their identity weakens. This reassurance as to one's identity depends very much upon being a member of a group where one has certain tasks to perform, certain roles in regard to the life of this group. Here one can see one's self constantly reflected, as it were, in the eyes of someone else; so that you know who you are because the other people know who you are, and you can tell from their reaction to you who you are.

It is very hard to tease these things apart in a normal naturally occurring situation, because they go on silently. But the way in which you find out about them is when this natural situation is upset. For instance, people who have studied the reactions of displaced persons, of immigrants, of people who leave their home and family and move to other places, discover that many of these people show disorders which are based upon the weakening of their confidence in their own identity.

I suppose that most people have felt this to some small extent in their own life. When you leave town and you go to a strange place you get a 'stranger' feeling. If you introspect, you discover that what this amounts to is that you are not too certain of who you are, or what you do, or what you should do, and you feel rather lost. Now, that feeling of being rather lost is a normal manifestation. We have all experienced this to some extent; but if you multiply it many times over you can imagine what it feels like to be someone who is entirely out of his normally existing group and in an entirely strange situation.

One finds this confusion also in patients who have certain disorders of personality. One of the characteristic disorders which one sees very often is a disorder of the capacity to know one's own identity. These people are always behaving in a completely different way in different circumstances, and they never feel that they have any consistent identity. Characteristically, what these people very often do is to do things to other people in order to create certain impressions, so that the other people should then reflect back to them that they are people of a certain kind. I had one patient who was doing this the whole time. He would go out and talk to different people and he was always acting some kind of part in order that they should look at him and see who he was, and then they would have some reaction to this, and from their reaction he would know who he was.

This particular rather complicated interchange is one of the reasons why from a mental health point of view it is important to be a member of a stable group, in which you have certain jobs to do and certain prescribed ways of behaving, so that you are constantly reminded of the fact that the other people look at you in a certain way. Clearly, when I talk about a small group here, I am mainly referring to the most characteristic small group of this kind, namely the family. It is interesting that if you ask someone the question, 'Who are you? What is your identity?', he answers, 'I am Tom Jones.' What is Tom Jones? Tom is his given name, and Jones is his family name; and who gave him his given name? His family. So Tom Jones is telling you, 'Who am I? I am a member of the Jones family, and I am Tom, the one who was given this name by Mr. and Mrs. Jones to differentiate him from the other children.' And so when you ask someone what his identity is, he focuses his identity on his membership of his little family group, and on his position in the group, which was determined by what the other people called him.

This is one of the most important theoretical points that Ackerman (1958) makes, namely, the significance of the way in which you fit into the family, and the way in which the family deals with you in regard to determining your identity.

Personal achievement and recognition. The last need which I wish to mention, though it is not nearly as fundamental as the others is the need which we have at least in our culture, and it varies from culture to culture, for personal achievement in material and spiritual matters. This is clearly a very much culturally determined need because, in certain cultures, people do not have this need for individual achievement. They may have a need for being, they may have a need to be happy, to be contented, to be a dutiful son, and to be a good father. As we begin to recite the things they have a need to be, we discover that many of them are included within the framework of being a person in an appropriate position within the family group and within the larger social group. But in our culture, we have a need for individual personal achievement; and we have a need not only to achieve ourselves, but also for the recognition of this achievement by others. So here again we have a situation with interpersonal implications. When you achieve something, it is not sufficient that you know it, but once again, you need the reassurance that someone else sees that you achieve it. You see this very well with children. They are constantly asking for 'attention', which means that you have to notice that they have done something. You find it also with grown-up people.

Anyone in an administrative position soon realizes that his administrative subordinates are not usually just content with accomplishing something, but they require fairly frequent recognition from their administrative superiors, that in fact these people recognize that they have achieved what they have. Any of you in administrative positions will notice that if you do not recognize in quite explicit form, and at regular intervals, the achievement of your subordinates, after a relatively short time the subordinates begin to get rather confused, which is another manifestation of this identity problem.

Now all these needs have to be satisfied to a greater or lesser extent in one's interaction in social situations. Some of the needs can be gratified in work groups as I have just mentioned. But the family is, in our culture, the main social institution which satisfies most of these needs and produces an appropriate balance between one and the other. In addition to the family and work groups, there are religious groups and social groups, etc., each of them emotionally meaningful clusters of interpersonal relationships in which each of us is involved. We have a certain number of needs, and we divide our search for their gratification among these various groups. But you will find that in our culture a major proportion of the needs are focused upon the core social grouping of the family.

Within the family we discover that these needs are not all

focused on one person. As you look at the individual's interactions with his family from this point of view, you discover that he has a repertoire of needs, and he divides them among the different people in the family; and the family group is so organized that the interaction of the various roles results in the gratification of most of the needs of the various family members. So here there is a complicated situation of a variety of needs focused on this family group, focusing differently upon each person in the family group, and the family group arranged in such a way that it satisfies the needs of the different people.

Now what happens if a family, which has been operating satisfactorily in this way, becomes disturbed, for instance by one member being removed. In those circumstances, it is necessary for the other people in the family to alter their roles so that they take up the slack. They must step into the place of the person who is missing. In certain circumstances, this is very difficult or impossible, and here I want to return to a question raised in Chapter 4; what happens in a family where one of the major actors in the drama is missing, for instance, the father? You may try, on the one hand, to bring someone else into the family circle to occupy that particular status and role. It is clear from what I have said above that there is possibly another way of dealing with this problem. Since a person's total needs are not entirely focused inside the family, an alternative would be to try to satisfy needs that cannot be satisfied inside the family through other networks outside the family. There are various ways of bringing a man into the house; maybe there is the possibility of invoking the aid of a school-teacher, a boy scout leader, or a minister of religion. Thinking on these lines, I am moving out of the family system and saying that because that certain need is not being satisfied by the provision of someone within the family system, it might be advisable to send the individual outside the family into some other social circle to find someone who will be able to satisfy the particular need.

Perhaps it might be as well now to summarize what I have said so far. I have talked about psychological needs, and I have pointed out that their satisfaction in the appropriate proportion is necessary for mental health. I have implied that the family is to be regarded from this point of view as a small social group of people bound together by meaningful emotional bonds, so that they focus their needs upon each other, and so that they satisfy each other's needs. If this process works satisfactorily it is conducive to the mental health of all the family members. If there are disorders in the relationships of people, in their ability to perceive each other's needs, in their respect for each other's needs, and in their ability to satisfy each other's needs, you are apt to get difficulty; and if the family gets disrupted by the removal of one or other member at the wrong time in its life cycle, then you are also apt to run into trouble. This, then, is one important aspect in the functioning of the family in regard to the mental health of its members.

There is another function to which I have alluded many times in the past chapters. That is the importance of the family during crises. As we have said repeatedly, when a person is in a crisis situation, when he is facing an important problem, which to begin with he has not the capacity to solve by the use of his ordinary repertoire of problem-solving methods, and he gets upset, one important factor that will determine the outcome will be the nature of his family's reaction to this situation.

Our hypothesis is that an individual facing a crisis situation is more likely to emerge in a mentally healthy way if during the crisis the family adds its strength to his, supports him, and does this in a way that is conducive to effective problem-solving, than if his family either does not add its strength to his, or if it presses him to move in an unhealthy direction.

A Study of Families in Crisis

In order to approach the testing of this hypothesis, we have been doing some preliminary work at Harvard School of Public Health in studying families where there is a crisis situation. I emphasize that this is preliminary work, and that the results which I am going to report are impressions gained during the reconnaissance and pilot stages of the research.

146

In this research[1] we have made contact with a random sample of lower-class and lower middle-class white and Negro families just after the onset of a crisis; and we have chosen as our primary crisis the reactions of the families to the birth of a premature baby. We have also studied the reactions of families to the birth of a congenitally deformed baby, although we have not collected as many cases in that category, and we have studied the reactions of families to a family member being diagnosed as having tuberculosis. But our main group is a group of cases of families where a premature baby has been born, and it is about these that I am going to talk. Our research team included a nurse, two other psychiatrists, a sociologist, an anthropologist, and a psychologist. This group of workers teamed up with the public health nurses in a city health centre in Boston. These public health nurses, as part and parcel of their everyday work, have dealings with the families of premature babies. They are informed immediately by the hospital when a premature baby is born, and they go to the home in order to investigate whether it is suitable for the reception of the baby. They hear of the birth by means of a notification slip sent out by the hospital; and a copy of this comes to us; so that we get to know of the case at the same time. In this way we obtain a list of all the premature babies that are born within the geographical jurisdiction of the city health centre. It so happens that the health centre is situated among a population where the people are mainly of lower, or of lower-middle socio-economic class, about half and half Negro and white.

When we get this list of cases, we sample the list in a random manner. We do not choose ahead of time that we will deal with this case or that case on the basis of anything idiosyncratic in the case itself. When the nurse goes out on her first visit to the home, one of our workers goes with her. She introduces this worker to the family as 'one of the people who works in the health centre, who is interested in the problems of families who have premature babies'; and after she has done her part of the visit she turns the interview over to our worker, who then intro-

[1] This research has been financed by a grant from the Commonwealth Fund.

duces himself and tries to arouse the motivation of the family to allow him to come into the home about once a week for the next two or three months during an evening when the whole family is present, in order to talk with them about the problems that they are meeting in regard to this premature baby. He tells them that the purpose of the study is to learn more about the problems of dealing with premature babies, so that we can improve health services. Interestingly enough, the vast majority of people we talk to in this way are quite willing to co-operate in the study, although they realize that they will get no direct service themselves from our efforts.

We visit in the evening or some other time when it is most convenient to see all the members of the family. We also invite some of them individually to come up to our office to talk to us. For people, especially when they are talking to you in their own home and in the presence of other members of the family, will not talk about certain things. There are certain topics which are not talked about, and which are not even thought very consciously about; but if you take someone right out of the home into a unique situation like a health department office or a psychologist's office, he is able to lay down many of his usual defences in this strange situation, and is able to discuss matters that he would not ordinarily talk or think about.

I am reporting on findings in about thirty cases, all of whom were studied intensively for about eight to ten interviews, at weekly intervals. These families were studied continuously through the period when the baby was in the hospital and the mother was home, which was usually when we made our first contact, because the mother was usually home by the time we got the first notification of the prematurity; then during the phase when the baby came home; and for at least six weeks afterwards. There was usually a follow-up visit a month or two later. Each interview was carefully recorded. In our earlier contacts, we used portable tape-recorders, but later we decided that it was not worth the time and effort involved, and we could record the kind of thing in which we were interested in a reasonably objective way without this device. As soon as the worker returned from a visit he sat down and wrote the record while the issues were fresh in his memory.

My main report is based on the findings in only twelve of these cases. These cases we separated from the whole thirty for the following reason. We wanted to find out the relationship between the way the family behaved during the crisis period and the mental health outcome. But here we struck one of the main rocks of this kind of mental health research. No one in his right mind would suggest that at the end of two to three months after the premature baby has come home we are likely to see any significant alteration in the psychiatric picture of the family, except in very special circumstances. That is to say, we imagine that an unhealthy resolution will lead to mental disorder, not now, but maybe in a year or two or three. So what can we use as our consequent variable, as our criterion of whether the family has done well or has not done well? This is a very general problem in this kind of research. What we did was to pay attention to our original theoretical model. You will remember that the original formulation is that the family is important for the mental health of its members (*a*) because it satisfies their needs, and (*b*) because in a crisis situation it supports the individual members. We therefore decided to use one of these as the antecedent variable of our equation, and the other manifestation as the consequent variable. In other words we investigated the effect of different patterns of dealing with crisis upon changes in the degree of satisfaction of needs within the family circle. So our consequent criterion variable is, 'Is there any change during the duration of the crisis in the way the family satisfies the psychological needs of its members?' Those families which appeared to be satisfying the psychological needs of their members less well at the end of the crisis than before, we called the *Unhealthy Outcome* group. Those families which, at the end of the crisis, appeared to satisfy the needs of the members as well as, or better, than before, we called the *Healthy Outcome* group.

Now, of the thirty cases that we studied intensively, we discovered that only in twelve could we say definitely that they were clearly Unhealthy Outcome cases, or clearly Healthy Outcome cases. The others were intermediate or indeterminate. We took only the extreme cases. There were five cases on one side, and seven on the other; and we contrasted these two polar groups with each other in regard to how they dealt with the crisis problem.

We took records of the two groups of cases and we examined them and we tried to isolate what you might call 'ideal types' of response, generalized pictures of response, which differentiated one group from the other. I will now describe the very general pictures we found by this analysis.

In the Healthy Outcome cases there was effective leadership on the part of one or both parents; good communication among family members; clear role assignments that appeared appropriate to the capacity of members, in other words no one was asked to do something that he was intellectually or physically incapable of doing, at least not for more than a very short time; and flexibility of role assignment, that is to say, the job that each person had to do was not always the same, it was flexible, so that if one person was weakened or absent, another could step in and do the job.

In the Unhealthy Outcome cases, on the other hand, there was poor and inconsistent leadership. The parents disagreed as to dominance; they could not decide who was the boss at any particular time or – very interesting from the mental health point of view – they abdicated their leadership role in crisis and parentified their children, that is to say, instead of the parent being the leader and supporting the children in the family, the parent became ineffectual and leaned on the children, so that one or the other of the children was forced into taking the leadership role. Communication was poor, messages were often not passed on or were distorted. Role assignments were not clear or were inappropriate; people were asked to do things that they were incapable of doing, and people did not know what they were supposed to do. Role assignment was rigid. Important jobs were not done if the person usually doing them was weak or absent; for instance, if the mother was away or if she was

150

tired, the house became dirty and the meals were not prepared. No one else stepped into the breach.

In dealing with a premature baby, the main individual handling the problem, the main victim of the crisis, as it were, is the mother; but other people also have jobs to do in regard to the premature baby. In regard to the help afforded the individual facing the problem, we found that in the Healthy Outcome group, the family culture and traditions and values emphasized the importance of facing trouble with open eyes, striving to learn the details of the problem, keeping the problem constantly in awareness, and trying to modify the outcome by individual and group action. In other words, in the Healthy Outcome families it was the custom in the family that, if you had a problem, you looked at it, you thought about it, you worried about it, and you went out looking for information about it. In these families, the customs of the family meant that, in regard to the premature baby, there was constant visiting, asking questions, and trying to find out about it. If the people in the hospital did not tell them what the answers were, they went around asking their friends who had had premature babies, or they tried to read about it. The individual was urged to conform to this pattern, and he was helped in this fact-finding, in his planning, and in his actions, by the rest of the family. So in cases where the wife was not too keen on visiting the baby, the other members of the family would urge her to go, or the others would go and get the information and tell her, or someone would phone up, and so on. There was a general scurrying around in these families to find out what a premature baby is, what causes it, and what you do about it.

The family also encouraged the individual to verbalize his negative feelings that were provoked by the danger and frustration of the crisis, and helped him keep these feelings within bearable bounds. For instance, anxiety was respected. It was recognized that family members were anxious, and this was greeted with sympathy by the other members. The anxiety was lowered by occasional reassurance. When someone in the family became too anxious, the rest of the family would calm him down. Guilt was relieved; the mother would be encouraged to say something like, 'It was all my fault.' Then the husband would say to the wife, 'Well, now, look here, you did as much as you could do, and it can't be your fault that this has happened.' Depression was shared, such as the depression of the mother when she could not see her baby. In certain of the hospitals in the Boston area there are quite high barriers between parents and their premature babies. The woman who had expected to bring home a baby came home on her own bereft of her baby, and she was depressed and miserable. The rest of the family would share her misery and say, 'We feel miserable too.' Blaming others was discouraged. Blaming is a defence against guilt by what we call projection; along the lines of, 'It isn't my fault at all, it is his fault.' This led to anger at the hospital authorities, at the doctors and nurses, 'If the doctor and nurses had not done this or that, I wouldn't have delivered the baby so soon. They are responsible.' When these reactions were voiced, they were always quickly counteracted by the other members of the family. They would say, 'Well now, look, after all, the nurses there are doing all they can and surely they are very busy, and they haven't got time to talk to you, but after all it is not their fault that it is a premature baby.'

Next, the individual was helped to concentrate his energy on the problem by having some of his other family tasks taken over by the others. For instance, in these families husbands often did the housework usually done by the wife; and when the baby came home, the husband often took his turn at attending to the baby. The important aspect here is that this help was offered in a collaborative and willing manner. You will observe in a moment the contrast in the Unhealthy Outcome group. In the Healthy Outcome group the individual who was being helped was never made to feel that he was imposing on the other's generosity. There was an absence of sufferance and charity. The help was given in an ego-supportive way. When the husband helped the wife, or when the children helped the mother, they did it willingly, and they did it usually with some kind word. If you keep this in mind, you will notice the contrast in a moment.

152

Next, the family was sensitive to the state of well-being of the individual facing the brunt of the stress. When he became emotionally or physically fatigued, the others encouraged a rest period. For instance, the wife was urged to go to sleep, or to go out to the movies or to some other recreation, or to take a rest. 'You've been doing too much, you're worn out. Why don't you lie down?' This encouragement was accompanied by the offer to take over the job of caring for the premature baby for a while. On the other hand, and this is equally important, after an appropriate period of respite, there was a call back to arms. The woman was not allowed just to go on coasting along or forgetting about the problems; she was usually soon called back, 'Come back to work now, you've had enough rest.' The family would not permit prolonged abdication. They did not allow anyone just to give up the problems, there was a constant stimulation, 'Now come on, we've got to face it together.' This was the Healthy Outcome group.

In the Unhealthy Outcome cases the family culture encouraged the denial and avoidance of unpleasant reality issues. It encouraged magical wishful thinking, and it encouraged undue early resignation in the face of difficulties. Common slogans in these families were, 'Don't worry, and all will be well' or, 'Don't trouble trouble, and trouble won't trouble you.' There was also the feeling in these families that one's own actions are not likely to affect the outcome of a crisis. 'What will happen will happen.' In line with these values, the family encouraged the individual beset by difficulties to avoid and to deny them, and not to investigate the situation too closely, or to preoccupy himself with plans for problem-solving. It was quite interesting in these families to see that there was no hurrying or scurrying to look at the baby. They hardly looked at the premature baby at all. They did not go asking their friends what to do about this premature baby, and they did not read about it. (I would just emphasize here that there was no difference from a socio-economic or ethnic point of view between the two groups of cases. In other words, these differences I am describing were not due to the fact that one group was heavily loaded with lower-class people, and the other with middle-class people, nor were the Negroes in one group and the whites in the other.)

Any verbalization of negative feelings by the individual was received with discomfort by the family, and attempts were made to end it quickly by massive and non-reality-based reassurance, and by encouraging him to blame others for his troubles. If the woman began to say how miserable she was, and how anxious she was, and to express concern about what might happen to the baby, the others would quickly say, 'No, the baby will be all right; there is nothing to worry about; everything is going to be fine,' or, 'It is the hospital's fault, it was those damn nurses, those young nurses, they are no good at all, they are probably students; and the doctors, they are all foreigners, you can't speak to them.' If there was any verbalization of negative feeling by the individual it was received with discomfort by the family, and it was stopped. People were not allowed in these families to express anxiety, to voice personal guilt, and to talk about their feelings of depression. If they tried to do so, they were stopped rather quickly by quick reassurance, and the statement that 'everything will be all right' or, as I have said, by turning the blame quickly on to outside people. Anything negative led to hostility toward outside people.

There was often no allowance made in the family circle for an individual to preoccupy himself with these crisis problems. He was not relieved of his other duties in the household. For instance, the husband and the other children continued to demand that the mother should do all her housework as before, despite the fact that at that moment she was worn out and depressed because of worrying about the baby in the hospital; or when the premature baby came home and she had the job of taking care of him and she was getting tired out, they continued to demand that she do what she was supposed to do. The family showed no obvious awareness of the individual's emotional or physical fatigue, and there was no encouragement to rest, apart from the overall fostering of abdication. They appeared to say, 'There is no problem, so you do not have to worry.' And this encouragement to abdication appeared to be mainly motivated by not wanting to be faced by signs of trouble in the family circle. When the individual did rest, there was no call back to arms. In other words, someone who wanted to avoid a problem was not stimulated by the others to come back and face it.

If the individual was obtrusively failing on some job in the house because of fatigue, someone else in these families sometimes did take over the task, but not in an ego-supporting manner. This was done usually by elbowing the individual out of the way in a spirit of condescending charity, or in a criticizing and belittling manner. We were very much impressed by the way certain husbands in this group, who noticed after a time that their wives were really falling down in taking care of the baby, would push the woman aside in a quite rivalrous way and say something belittling like, 'What a lousy mother you are. I can do the job better myself.' He would then change the baby, and would show during the care of the baby that he was a better mothering person than she was. Now, he was apparently helping by changing the baby, but the effect of this was to reduce her strength rather than to increase it, because what she felt was, 'He is showing that I am no good.' This contrasted markedly with the husbands in the other group, who, when they did the same thing, did it in such a way as to make the mother feel that her husband loved her, and was sacrificing something for her. When you talked to a woman in the Healthy Outcome group about her husband, she would talk in admiration about how he was showing such initiative, and how she had not expected that he would be capable of doing this, 'What a good husband he is, he even takes care of the baby in this way, and he does it beautifully. You ought to see him feed the baby.' The women in the Unhealthy Outcome group would make hostile remarks such as, 'Some man he is, he's always running after the baby. He feeds the baby as though he is a woman!' The reason they spoke in this way was that as far as they were concerned, this was an active rivalry situation between them. They were being pushed out of their role by their husbands. So that the net result of this 'help' was a weakening rather than a strengthening of the individual.

Finally, in the Unhealthy Outcome cases, the tension of the crisis in the family group appeared often to be lowered at the emotional expense of some particular family member. It was usually a child who suffered, a child who was essentially the vulnerable member of the family. For instance, we noticed that a toddler might be scapegoated and become the target for hostility of a parent who appeared to be trying to escape feelings of guilt; and these feelings of guilt, as far as we could tell, were based upon irrational fantasies of responsibility for the premature birth. You would notice that in these families the parents would first of all show manifestations of feeling guilty and you would get some hints in talking to them that they thought they had caused the prematurity. Not infrequently the woman would feel she had done it, because she thought she had bumped herself, or she had run around, or something like that. Not infrequently they had had intercourse the night before, or two nights before, and the doctor had said this was not permitted, or the doctor had not said anything, but they themselves believed that it was not permitted, and this was what had caused the prematurity. And after quite a short time, you would find that they were beginning to pick on one of the children. Usually a toddler would be the victim because, at this particular stage, he would probably be demanding more attention as a reaction to feelings of deprivation, since the mother had been out of the home and the family was upset. So he would be making more demands, and they would start scapegoating him. In one case where they picked on a toddler the mother said, 'It was because of the nuisance he made while I was pregnant, and I had to carry him around, and that was what brought on the premature labour.' Instead of being hostile to the doctors and nurses, or instead of being hostile to themselves, the parents became hostile to one of the children, and thus relieved their feelings of guilt. Or the child may be emotionally exploited by neglect, through the diversion of parental attention on to the premature baby. Of course, the premature baby requires attention, but we found in certain cases that it was getting more attention than it needed; and this also seemed to be related to feelings of guilt; the reaction being, 'I have done you damage, therefore I will repair the damage by being especially careful about you.' This would seem to be an expiation of guilt. Now, two people were victimized by this: one, the premature baby itself because a premature baby needs attention, but it does not need over-attention, it does not need to be choked with cotton-wool; and, secondly, the other child was suffering.

In the Healthy Outcome cases, it was always clear that, however preoccupied the parents were with the presenting problem, they could always spare a side-glance for the rest of the family, and they were watching all the time what this one's needs were, and what that one needed; however preoccupied she was with the premature baby, the woman was always paying attention to her husband and to the other children, to make sure that as much as was possible they were not suffering.

In the Unhealthy Outcome cases, we also found another reaction – an older child becoming a displacement object for exaggerated anxiety stimulated by fantasies about the danger to the life of the baby. We were very much impressed in this case by the fact that the parents suddenly became very anxious about one of the other children. This child seemed perfectly all right, and yet they constantly worried about him. It appeared to be that their real worry was about the premature baby, but they could not worry about the premature baby because this was real worry, since the premature baby was, in fact, in danger; so they unconsciously chose to worry about the other child, who was not in danger. At some level they realized he was not, and so they could feel that all their worries were unreal. In all these cases, the toddler is cast into a new role in the family, which neglects his current needs and allows the other members to work out vicariously on him certain problems aroused by the crisis, which they have been unable to handle directly.

The disordered relationship which thus begins may have a clearly pathogenic effect on the toddler's development if it continues for any length of time. One thing which our studies so far have not shown is why in certain circumstances the other children are used in this way, as a method of solving the family problem, whereas in other cases they are not; and why under certain circumstances these children are used in this way only for a short time, whereas in other cases it leads to a continuing disordered relationship. Obviously, if a child is scapegoated only for a short time, he is not going to suffer very much; but if the scapegoating continues, it produces a gross distortion in the relationship between the parents and himself, and this certainly has pathogenic significance for his future mental health.

I think you will have noticed that the descriptions of these ideal types seem richer than you would expect from a dozen cases. The reason for this is that we have rounded out the picture by using some other cases which were not in our two groups, when we noticed in these other cases certain reactions which seemed similar to the reactions in the twelve cases. We have thus amplified the picture a bit, which is perhaps not scientifically valid. But at this particular stage we do not want to narrow our scope by too stringent reliance on strict research design. We are still at the stage of developing hunches and hypotheses, and so we have been using our intuition, and we have been looking at all our cases in a clinical anecdotal way, although the main out-lines of the picture definitely came from the comparison of our two polar groups.

This may give you some idea of the kind of work that is involved in this type of research. It is not at all easy to do this. It will take us a number of years before we come out with any reliable picture, but it is possible already to see how, from the kind of observations we have described, we can classify the family of a premature baby as being towards the unhealthy pole or towards the healthy pole. If the family's responses to crisis seem to be towards the healthy pole, we can be pleased and merely hold a watching brief; but if the responses seem to be towards the unhealthy pole, we can identify this as a case which merits preventive intervention. The study also affords some hints as to the type of intervention. This would consist of trying to move the behaviour of the family by whatever means possible from the unhealthy pattern over to the healthy pattern.

DISCUSSION

Question: Was intervention used in those cases which appeared to be moving towards the unhealthy pole?

Answer: Not by design. But clearly when you go week after week into a family in crisis, you are certainly altering the picture. The very fact that we are talking with these people about their feelings and about what they are doing, and especially the kind of questions that we ask, certainly alter the picture, although our interviewers were very skilled and were doing their best not to suggest anything. Our intervention probably affected all the cases and moved the whole sample over to the healthy side. So our unhealthy cases were possibly less unhealthy as a result of our being there and talking to them in this way.

Of course, I cannot rule out that some may have been hindered by our presence, in particular, Negroes of lower socio-economic class may have been burdened by a middle-class white interviewer who kept coming in and badgering them when they were busy trying to deal with their problems in their own traditional way. But there was no way of avoiding this apart from getting a cloak of invisibility. David Shakow at the National Institute of Mental Health has thought of installing a television camera in the corner of a room in the family's home and recording everything that takes place. I do not know whether he has managed to do it. But even that, of course, will alter what is going on. So there is no way of not altering the situation; the only thing is that we did our best not to alter anything in a specific way; and we certainly did our best never to intervene in any directed way to try to alter the pattern from one kind to another.

This was controlled by the fact that the interviewer was supervised by other members of the team. The records were carefully read by other people. If anyone seemed to show any signs of intervening, this was drawn to his attention. On one occasion I remember, the interviewer, who was a social worker, had a terrible time. He felt this family was ruining one of the children, and he just could not stand by and see it happen. I spent about two hours with him one day, and effectively stopped him from intervening. It was a good job I did this, because in that particular case what happened about a week later was that the family themselves spontaneously altered their way of behaving in a way that neither of us could have foreseen. If he had intervened as he had wished, it would have obscured the picture.

Now, you may say there is an ethical problem involved here. We are going into the homes of families, and we see things that seem hazardous. Why don't we intervene? Well, I do not feel guilty about it because even after three years' work I can only give you a very tentative picture of the two extreme patterns; and I am still not certain that they are correct.

The families were being carried by a public health nurse, who continued to deal with them all the time that we were studying them. And she was doing whatever she could in the circumstances to help the family deal with their problems. We took care not to influence her way of handling her cases, so she handled the family's problems in her traditional way. One of the things that we were investigating which I have not discussed was whether the traditional way of functioning of the caretaking agents was helpful or not, and whether we can find some other way that they might operate in a more helpful manner in these crisis cases. And so we did our best not to alter what the hospital was doing, and what the public health nurse was doing. They were free to go ahead and do as much for this family as they would have done for any other family. As a matter of fact, and again this is a distorting element, it seemed that a public health nurse who was carrying one of our study families undoubtedly paid more attention to this particular family than she did to her usual caseload. You can be sure of that, since there were case conferences at which she would have to report. So that, again, the whole group was probably being moved in a healthy direction. I suppose that there were fewer cases in our unhealthy group than there would have been if we had had a cloak of invisibility and could have gone in and seen what the families did entirely without our intervention.

Question: Was there any difficulty in dividing the cases into the two polar groups?

Answer: With many of them it was difficult, and so we excluded them from the analysis. It does not appear to be difficult to place the extreme cases into one group or the other. There were certain cases where it was clear to everyone. Incidentally, I did not give all the details of our research design, but we went through a whole process of controls in dividing the cases up. We removed the names from the records and removed the signs of whether it was a Healthy or an Unhealthy Outcome case, and then we submitted the record to different judges and asked them to define the family reactions to crisis. We gave the outcome parts of the records to another judge and asked him to classify the outcome. We have done our best to avoid being biased by classifying a case in the Unhealthy Outcome group because we recognized in it unhealthy ways of dealing with problems. In certain cases, there is no doubt at all, and different judges will come up with the same answer so that you can place the families neatly at either one pole or the other. With many other cases, it is hard to know. Also, if in a family some of the members behaved in one way during a crisis, and others in another way, it was rather difficult to determine the predominant family pattern. In regard to the outcome variables, this was no problem. If any single member of the family related in a worse way to any other member of the family at the end of the crisis, that family was placed in the Unhealthy Outcome group. And the only people in the Healthy Outcome group were families where every single member appeared to be relating in as healthy a way to every other member at the end as at the beginning. So in the Healthy Outcome group we can be fairly confident, but in the Unhealthy Outcome group there were all gradations. In one family there may have been only one relationship that appeared to be disordered; in other families there were many relationships that appeared to be disordered.

Question: Did you follow up your families to discover the eventual result of crisis changes?

Answer: I think we are likely to do some follow-up to see whether the Unhealthy Outcome group does in fact eventually show psychiatric disturbance in any of its members that did not exist before. But the numbers of cases were so small that, if you wanted to design a study to do that kind of thing, it would have to be of a different nature. You would have to design a more extensive study with larger numbers of people, where you would not have to go into all the intensive interviewing that we did. In these thirty cases, each record is about three inches thick. Every interview of an hour to two hours has maybe fifteen to twenty typewritten pages of notes, so there is a great deal of work involved, which means that you can only see a very small number of cases. In order to satisfy ourselves on the point you raise we would use another design.

Question: What factors appeared to predispose families to handle crisis problems in a healthy or unhealthy way?

Answer: There are many, many factors which we did not take into account. They were not important, however, for our precise hunch. We were not, in this research, particularly interested in what are the predisposing factors to unhealthy problem-solving as compared to healthy problem-solving. What we were interested in was a current description of what you see in a family during a crisis, and how you can tell whether it is going to come out healthy or unhealthy.

We had a limited focus in this study. In future studies we intend to deal with the question you have asked, since it is obviously important.

REFERENCE

ACKERMAN, NATHAN (1958). *The Psychodynamics of Family Life.* New York : Basic Books.

CHAPTER 6

The Role of the Nurse in Maternal and Child Care

An important trend in present-day mental hygiene is away from the concentration of effort on early diagnosis and treatment of individuals suffering from emotional disorder, and toward the goal of identifying and altering the sets of circumstances which might lead to such a disorder. Our attention has shifted from pathology in the patient to the pathological factors in the environment.

We recognize that the most significant area of a person's environment in relation to his mental health is the complexity of emotional inter-relationships which focus on him. These relationships are most significant during his early formative years, but remain important throughout his life.

In any community, certain individuals have roles which make them key people for the mental health of many others. If these individuals have disturbed relationships with their fellows, they may exert a pathogenic effect on their emotional life, and may be likened to 'carriers' of mental ill-health similar to the 'carriers' of typhoid and other infectious diseases.

Preventive psychiatry is attempting today to identify such key people who are disturbed and have disturbing relationships, and to ameliorate their distorted attitudes in order to prevent their pathogenic effect in the community. It is also studying the circumstances which produce such disturbed relationships in order to prevent these people from becoming mental-ill-health 'carriers'.

163

This work is being undertaken in the hope that the further back the pathogenic process can be traced, the simpler will be the factors involved and the less costly will be their treatment.

In considering the circumstances which produce disturbed relationships and also the conditions under which these have their maximum pathogenic effect, the concept of emotional crisis has become important. Whatever their prevailing emotional relationships with their fellows, people are usually in a condition of emotional equilibrium. There is some stability in their mental life whether they are emotionally ill, or healthy, whether they are carriers of mental health or of ill-health. Under certain conditions, however, this balance of psychic forces is upset and for a period, often quite short, the person is in a state of emotional disequilibrium. At such times of crisis, a relatively small force acting for a short time may tip the balance either to one side or to the other, and once tipped over, a new stable equilibrium is obtained. Such a crisis may lead a key person to develop into a carrier of emotional ill-health. During the brief period of disequilibrium, a person may be more vulnerable to the pathogenic effect of a 'carrier'. But it is precisely at such crisis periods that the mental hygienist may operate most profitably by lending his emotional strength to the healthy side of the balance of psychic forces and, by the expenditure of minimal energy, produce fundamental changes in the attitudes of people. The goal of mental hygiene, therefore, is to identify crisis periods among important people in the community, and to ensure that they will emerge from these crises with healthy interpersonal relationships, so that they will not become carriers of mental ill-health.

Among these key people are parents, kindergarten teachers, other teachers, army officers, foremen in industry, and similar persons in charge of others. Here we will discuss the mother, who has been studied more than any of the others. Although she comes into contact with a smaller number of susceptible individuals, her influence for good or ill on her young children is probably the most potent environmental factor in their emotional development.

In studying the circumstances which produce a disturbed mother-child relationship and turn the mother into a carrier of emotional ill-health, we have learned that she goes through a period of increased susceptibility to crises which stretches from pregnancy through the lying-in period and into her child's first few years of life.

During pregnancy, the biological processes and their emotional impact stimulate the re-emergence of problems of her femininity and its association with her relationship to her own mother, which may have been only partially solved in the past. The general emotional crisis may also stir up any other personality weakness and lead to emotional disequilibrium. Problems for which solutions in the past were incomplete may be revived, giving opportunity now to find a better or a worse solution for them. Pregnancy, therefore, may lead to greater maturity and healthier relationships, or it may lead to the kind of pathogenic situation in which the expectant mother prepares to use the coming child as a partial solution for some of her problems. The danger is always present that she may relate to her child primarily on the basis of fulfilling her own need to solve those internal problems just mentioned. This type of relationship, likely to pervert the child's development, contrasts with a healthy mother-child relationship in which the mother reacts to her child primarily on the basis of her awareness of his needs and her attempt to satisfy them.

The emotional crises of pregnancy are produced mainly through stimulation by biological processes within the mother, but after the child is born and during his early years, similar crises may be produced because the mother is stimulated from without by her intimate association with him. As he passes through successive stages of instinctual development, this association stimulates the deepest layers of her personality structure, which were laid down when she was his age. Disequilibria similar to those occurring in pregnancy – with the same range of healthy or pathogenic outcomes – may be the result.

MENTAL HYGIENE ACTIVITIES DURING PREGNANCY
AND THE POSTPARTUM PERIOD

These considerations lead mental health workers to concentrate on programmes of mental hygiene supervision for the pregnant woman and the mother of young children, and the following types of activity have been among those found useful.

Ego Strengthening or general Support

This type of mental hygiene activity is nonspecific and is likely to be of some use in most cases. Regardless of the presence or absence of crises or of their types, the worker lends his emotional support to the patient, so that her balance of psychic forces is weighted down in the direction of health and maturity. This is accomplished by the worker actively expressing an attitude of human interest and an understanding of the mother as an individual with her own characteristics and idiosyncrasies, and by accepting her as she is.

This is a very concrete and practical kind of help, but it is hard to describe. The following examples may make it clearer.

A 31-year-old woman, after attending a sterility clinic for two years, was discharged from the clinic as a hopeless case, and she and her husband reconciled themselves with difficulty to a life of childlessness. The wife embarked on a professional career and they made elaborate plans to travel abroad in order to gain professional experience in different countries.

In the midst of these plans, the wife suddenly became pregnant and much to her own and her husband's surprise she reacted violently against it. Though she attended the prenatal clinic regularly and co-operated fully with her doctor, she was quite outspoken in her rejection of the pregnancy, and continued working until the last possible moment. She ascribed her resentment to the unexpectedness of this interruption of her carefully laid plans, saying, 'Previously when I did all I could to have a baby, I couldn't become pregnant,

166

and now when I have given it up and got going on something else, this comes along!'

The public health workers were very interested in the underlying psychological mechanisms, but they made no active attempt to uncover them. Instead, they built up a warm relationship with the woman and encouraged her to verbalize very freely her complaints against the unpredictability of her fate. Far from urging her to accept her lot with gratitude, they made their sympathy clear to her, and let her know that they understood her negative feelings, and that they accepted and respected her just as much as they did patients who were happy with their pregnancies. This support became all the more meaningful to her as month followed weary month, and her complaints and rebellion continued unabated. She was repeatedly reassured that this free expression of her hostility to the pregnancy cast no reflection on her capacities as a potential mother and she was supported in her hopes that when the baby would be born, her original positive attitude to motherhood would return.

Her negativism did not disappear until she went into labour. A day later when she put her son to her breast for the first time, she felt a sudden wave of motherliness sweep over her, and thereafter she behaved like any average mother who loves her child.

A 19-year-old girl had suffered since childhood from all kinds of anxieties and fears. When she became pregnant, these were intensified and in addition to her old fears of the dark, burglars, heart trouble, or dropping dead, she was terrified that her baby would die, would be born mentally defective, or be a monster or blind or crippled.

Whenever she came to the prenatal clinic, and during frequent home visits by the nurse, she was allowed to talk freely about her fears and she was listened to with patience and sympathy. She was not reassured directly but her anxiety usually lessened when she became aware that the worker, listening carefully to her horror stories, was in no way upset by them. She was much strengthened when she found that she wasn't laughed at, or told to pull herself together, but that she was accepted as she was – a weak and nervous girl struggling hard to cope with problems that most other people hardly bother about. Any signs of strength were noted and praised and the positive feelings she had about her husband and her pregnancy were recognized and appreciated. She was surprised to find that the workers continued to respect her despite all her nervousness, which she had previously felt to be in some way morally reprehensible, and her own self-respect was increased by this.

She bore her labour with what was for her great bravery but almost collapsed during the lying-in period when she was faced with the responsibility of caring for her baby. She was encouraged not to breast-feed and she was allowed to move very slowly in taking over the care of the child. During her first few weeks at home, the nurse made frequent visits and answered innumerable phone calls. She allowed the mother to be childishly dependent on her and accepted her very slow development toward ordinary material responsibility.

Little by little, this mother began to realize what she meant to her baby, who was so much more helpless than she, and whose satisfactory development soon began to bear witness to her maternal devotion. After the third or fourth month, the patient's fears lessened considerably and with her increasing pride in her motherhood, a characteristic maturing process became evident in her total personality.

It is hard in these and other cases to evaluate the importance of these techniques. A meaningful emotional relationship between the mother and an accepting, non-judging worker certainly helps to strengthen the ego-integrative forces in the mother's personality. Perhaps the chief significance of such a relationship lies in its insurance value – in case of a crisis, the mother can immediately borrow strength from the worker to whom she has become attached.

Mobilizing environmental Sources of Love and Support

The pregnant woman needs extra love just as much as she needs extra vitamins and protein. This is especially so in the last few months of pregnancy and during the nursing period. During pregnancy she often becomes introverted and passively dependent. The more she is able to accept this state, and the more love and solicitude she gets from the people around her, the more maternal she can be toward her child. Professional workers cannot give her the love she needs, but they can mobilize the members of her family, and especially her husband, to do so. In our culture, husbands and other relatives are often afraid of 'spoiling' the expectant mother and special efforts are needed to counteract this attitude.

A warm and sensitive young girl, married to a rather cold, intellectual, and shut-in man, showed many signs of insecurity throughout pregnancy. She sometimes talked of her longing to see her mother, to whom she was much attached, but who lived thirty miles away. Her husband was away at his job all day and most of the evening, so she had bought a pet dog to comfort her in her loneliness. The husband was told of his wife's increasing demands for signs of affection and said that he feared she was getting soft and childish. In a couple of short discussions, he was helped to ventilate his anxiety that she would become an emotional burden on him. He was then urged to spend as much time as possible at home and was reassured that her regressive passivity and increased demands for love were quite normal manifestations of pregnancy. He was advised to make special efforts to demonstrate his love as concretely as possible, both by personal attentions and by helping with the housework. He was also supported in a plan to buy a small secondhand car so that his wife could visit her mother. His relations with his mother-in-law were cool, but when he understood the importance of providing his wife with as much love and affection as possible, he readily agreed to invite his mother-in-law to stay with them during the last week of pregnancy and the first few weeks after his wife returned with the baby.

The young mother's response to these simple measures was gratifying, and she made a surprisingly smooth adjustment to the early stages of nursing and caring for her baby.

Anticipatory Guidance

This technique has been much described during recent years and will, therefore, receive only brief mention here. It is a valuable method of mobilizing the patient's strength beforehand so that she is able to meet a crisis situation more constructively. She is told in detail what to expect, and by imagining in advance what it might feel like, she is able to lower her anxiety level and to develop a readiness for a healthy reaction. It is worth stressing that the technique works best when the future events are described in greatest detail and when the patient is given a full opportunity to discuss her feelings and particularly her anxieties beforehand.

In order to use this method, the worker must know the usual physical and emotional changes of pregnancy, labour, and child development, and he must be able to formulate his predictions reassuringly and yet without slurring over possible sources of difficulty. Examples of topics which can usefully be discussed with every pregnant woman include the sudden unexplainable mood changes, the irritability and emotional lability, and the passivity, which are so frequent in pregnancy. Possible changes in feelings about sex activity should usually be discussed at an early stage with both husband and wife. Fears and superstitions about maternal impression, difficult labour, and congenital abnormalities of various types are rendered less troublesome if these worries have been mentioned earlier by the worker as being a very significant inheritance from past ages.

Educational preparation of the expectant woman for labour has been advocated principally by the devotees of natural childbirth. It is certainly not necessary to subscribe to this doctrine in order to realize the importance of this technique. There is little doubt that a woman who has been told exactly what to expect will have a smoother and less traumatic experience in labour than someone who has no idea of what is coming next and is therefore a prey to her morbid imagination.

Similarly a few short discussions ahead of time on breast-feeding will pay excellent dividends, apart from helping an ambivalent woman to come to a clear decision beforehand, whether or not to nurse her baby. One mother felt no real love for her baby until he was three weeks old. Up to that time, she was interested in him and felt sympathetic and protective, but no more so than toward any other baby. She was not at all disturbed by this, and made a satisfactory adjustment to breast-feeding because she had been explicitly warned that this lack of maternal feeling would probably occur as a temporary phenomenon. This is an extreme case, but delays of two to five days before the mother feels fully maternal are not at all unusual nor are they unnatural.

Help in specific Crises

Intervention directed toward ensuring a healthy outcome to an emotional crisis must operate at the time of the acute disequilibrium in order to achieve a maximum effect. The same effort applied after the acute phase is over will have less chance of changing the balance. For this reason it is important to learn to recognize the crises of pregnancy and the post-partum period and, if possible, to be alert to their prodromal signs so that they can be predicted and prepared for.

This is an area in which our knowledge is still very scanty, but the following examples serve to illustrate what is involved.

A woman who had been adapting fairly well to her pregnancy suddenly became tense and anxious in her seventh month. She complained of mental confusion and ineffectiveness. She gave a history of a disturbed relationship with her mother, who had suffered a psychotic breakdown when the patient was a young girl and had been in a mental hospital for a couple of years. In an interview with the psychiatrist, the patient described with much emotion how upset she had been when her mother was taken away, and also how she had had to act as mother to the rest of the family, and even to her mother for years after her discharge from the hospital. In connection with her own present upset, she said that she was having a desired pregnancy and had felt fine until a week previously, when she had begun to feel passive and useless. Despite all her efforts, she could not shake off this apathy and she was now tense and sleepless. She said she was happily married but was completely frigid and even had some dyspareunia.

The psychiatrist pointed out to her that her introversion and passivity were a natural reaction of her present stage of pregnancy, but that apparently she had become very frightened because this sudden change in her feelings reminded her of her mother, who had always been a passive and ineffectual creature. She then broke into violent weeping and said that she was afraid she was going mad like her mother. She was shown how she had made an irrational link between her passivity and her mother's illness and she was urged to try to let nature have its way with her and to try to enjoy the passivity, instead of fighting it, as a positive contribution to her pregnancy.

She was tremendously relieved and very grateful for this help. During the rest of the pregnancy she was seen regularly for short interviews in which the same advice was repeated and she became quite relaxed. She had an easy labour and made a fairly good adjustment to breast-feeding, but she required continued support during the first few months of motherhood to relieve her anxiety that she would fail as a mother. Interestingly enough, six months after the delivery, she reported that she was no longer frigid and that she was planning another baby.

This girl had a deep disturbance of personality, involving conflicts relating to her femininity based on traumatic experiences with her mother. Orthodox psychotherapeutic help would probably have been difficult and certainly a very lengthy affair. When the biological changes of pregnancy precipitated her into a state of passivity, it upset her previous emotional equilibrium, in which she had defended herself against identifying with the mother's femininity by always being active and dominant. At this strategic moment, it was possible to help her to realize that passivity and femininity were not dangerous, and that she could be a woman and a mother without suffering the fate of her own mother. This help – as is possible in many cases – did not entail the lengthy process of giving her insight into the origin of her difficulties.

Another woman, toward the end of her second pregnancy, began to express worries lest she give birth to an ugly girl. Her first child was a girl and was very pretty. She feared that the coming baby could not be as nice and would be bound to have a hard time. She herself had been a tomboy and her mother had favoured her older sister who was pretty and feminine. Earlier in the pregnancy she had related this information with little show of emotion, but as delivery date approached, she remembered with great vividness her childhood jealousy of her sister and her own feelings of inferiority and insecurity in regard to her mother's affection. She was encouraged to talk freely about those old problems and she was shown quite directly that she was preparing to identify her new baby with herself as the younger of two girls, and was worried lest she reject it in the same way she imagined her mother had rejected her. This kind of encouragement relieved much of her anxiety but it is impossible to say how effective the intervention was because she gave birth to a boy.

This case is very interesting because it shows the train of events leading to the use of a child to work out unsolved conflicts of the mother. It also shows how buried problems come to the surface during pregnancy, and hints at the ease with which they can be handled.

A primipara had a smooth and normal pregnancy but had a long and difficult labour and the baby suffered a left-sided facial paresis from forceps. The mother had a bladder injury and had to stay in bed with an indwelling catheter. For administrative reasons, the baby was cared for in a nursery on a different floor of the hospital from the mother. Because the mother was unable to see it for the first three days, she refused to believe that the baby had only a mild injury. Her tension was relieved when she was given a true picture of the diagnosis and was told that she was entitled to be depressed and was encouraged not to try to put on a bold face. She was also given supervision and supportive help during breast-feeding. During this contact she confessed that she had been blaming herself for the difficult labour and the baby's injury, feeling that she had not carried out all the instructions given her in the prenatal clinic, particularly in regard to stopping sexual intercourse at the thirty-fourth week. Her guilt in relation to this was relieved.

This is a typical example of the danger to the mother-child relationship of a bad start, and the way in which the reality of a birth injury rapidly becomes involved in guilty fantasies based on past conflicts.

A young music student was seen in the fourth month of her pregnancy. She seemed strangely anxious about the well-being of the foetus and spent a long time discussing the signs of quickening. She admitted that the pregnancy had been unplanned and unwanted. A month later she was still asking for reassurance that the foetus was alive and healthy, which caused the obstetrician to suspect that she had done something to try to terminate the pregnancy. He told her that young girls who are upset at becoming pregnant sometimes try to interfere with the course of nature, and asked her outright whether she had attempted abortion. With much emotion, she confessed that she had done so but that she had told nobody about it – not even her husband, who was a theology student and felt that abortion was a terrible sin. She came from a religious family and they, too, would be upset if they found out what she had done. Now she felt terribly guilty and was sure that she had injured the baby. She felt she might have killed it, or at least if it lived to be born, it would be a monster of some kind. The obstetrician made no attempt to hide the fact that he felt she had done wrong, but by his tone of voice and by his continued interest he made her realize that her feelings of guilt were very much exaggerated. Opening up the subject and giving her the chance to share her secret offered her tremendous relief and when he felt that he had lessened her guilt feelings sufficiently, he then reassured her in regard to her anxieties that she had injured the baby. The obstetrician's simple but timely intervention saved this girl not only from the further torture of pathological guilt and anxiety, but from a probable disorder of her relationship with the child.

We have come to recognize that a failed attempt at abortion is a potent cause of a peculiarly pathogenic disorder of mother-child relationship. The mother typically shows great guilt in her handling of the child, feeling that she had previously attempted to murder him. She is tremendously anxious about his health, fearing that she must have injured him in some way, and by coddling and overprotection she manages to make him into a weakling, whom she takes from doctor to doctor for all kinds of treatments. She feels that this sickly creature who makes such demands on her time is the punishment for her crime. Often she regards him as the visible sign of her own badness and behaves quite cruelly to him, symbolically castigating her own sin in him.

Such children often appear in child guidance clinics with distorted personality structures. At this stage, it is hard to do anything for them and it is no consolation to the psychiatrist to trace the history of the disturbed mother-child relationship back to its origin in the traumatic incident of early pregnancy and to realize that a few sessions of simple treatment at that time would probably have prevented the subsequent sad development.

An Approach to Community Mental Health

Has the nurse a specialized function in this field of mental hygiene? She is a general practitioner among the many specialists who operate in maternal and child care – obstetricians, paediatricians, nutritionists, psychiatrists, psychologists, and social workers; she must know something of each of these specialties, and yet she is not competent to operate independently in any of them. She knows this and so does the patient, which is bound to make the nurse feel rather insecure. The competent nurse must know the boundaries and limitations of her work, but this insecurity may lead to the defence of denying her limitations, and trying to operate in the area of one of the specialists. Has she then no specialized function of her own? I feel that the answer to this question is very definitely in the affirmative.

The nurse's specialized function arises from her very special position in relation to her patient, and this is a role which is not open to any of the other specialists, except under atypical conditions.

The chief characteristic of this position is closeness.

Closeness in Space

The nurse goes into the patient's home, and in the hospital she remains at her bedside. She penetrates physically into the patient's environment.

Closeness in Time

The nurse's contact with the patient can be constant and continuous. She can make home visits throughout pregnancy; she is constantly present during labour and the lying-in period and when the mother returns home she can follow her there. It is not too difficult administratively to keep the number of nurses dealing with one patient at a minimum, and thus provide a unitary link right through the period under discussion. Apart from the importance of this in building up a supportive emotional relationship, its chief significance is that the nurse may often be actually present throughout a crisis situation.

Sociological Closeness

The traditional role of the nurse makes the patient regard her as being on the same status level as herself. In the professional relationship the patient feels that the other specialists are high above her in status; she regards them as parent-figures, but on this scale she considers the nurse a sibling figure. This means that communication is free and easy and involves little tension. She feels that the nurse speaks her language. There is no need to put on a show in front of her and she is not afraid to ask questions. In many countries this sibling role of the nurse is symbolized by calling her 'Sister'. She is traditionally not just an ordinary sister, but a specially wise sister – an older sister with experience and one who is interested in helping.

Psychological Closeness

Linked with the sociological closeness, which is based on the patient's perception of the nurse, is the fact that the nurse maintains less psychological distance than other professionals in treating her patients. She involves herself more freely, and uses herself more directly in a more unsophisticated and less rigid way, and with the use of fewer formalized psychological techniques. This human closeness is reciprocated by the patients, who show their feeling of freedom and ease by rapidly building up a trusting relationship.

I feel that this closeness is unique among the professional workers who are in contact with the mother and young child. The fundamental role of the wise sister, who is on the spot in time of trouble, gives the possibility of a unique and specialized function to the nurse. It is an important heritage, which must be jealously guarded, for if it is lost, the specialized mental hygiene functions of the nurse will be lost with it.

MENTAL HYGIENE FUNCTIONS OF THE NURSE

Case-finding

The nurse has the broadest contact with the mother and her human and physical environment. She can make her observations and collect her information when the people concerned are not on their guard and putting on a show. Moreover, she is frequently present when the members of the family are together, so that she can actually observe their interactional behaviour. This may throw a quicker and truer light on their interpersonal relations than hours of history-taking. This allows the nurse to specialize in identifying crisis situations, and in recognizing environmental circumstances that are hazardous to the interpersonal relationships of the patient and her family.

Initiation of Motivation

Having recognized a situation that is a mental health hazard, the nurse has an essential role in arousing the individual's motivation to seek the right professional help. In this work, since we are operating in a field in which symptoms often do not exist as a stimulus to seek help, and one in which the family members usually do not feel a need to involve themselves, the problem of motivation, which in the therapeutic setting is relatively simple, here becomes complicated and difficult. It is a problem which in certain cases may make the biggest demands on the skills of the psychiatrist, but the nurse must make the first move because it is her link with the mother or the relative which makes the initial interview possible.

Interpretation of the Patient to the Specialists

Routing the patient to the appropriate specialist is often the nurse's function, and is managed efficiently in most clinical settings. What is less well managed usually is the interpretation of the patient and her environment to the specialist sitting in his office. The nurse moves freely between the two worlds of patient and specialist. In each she should be regarded as an equal, and it should be her function to act as an emotional and intellectual bridge between them. Too often the wealth of information she has collected about a case remains locked inside her, and is not passed on to the other specialists. There are many reasons for this, but one thing is certain, and that is that both the nurse and the other professional workers ought to try to work out a more efficient method of ensuring this essential communication.

Interpretation of the Specialists to the Patient

It is the nurse's job not only to translate the words of the specialists into the patient's language, but also to unify the prescriptions of the different specialists and help the patient accept them as part of a coherent framework. It is interesting that at the present time she has much less difficulty dealing with interpretation in this than in the reverse direction.

Emotional Support

The special way in which the nurse gives emotional support has already been stressed – she gives assistance as a 'wise sister'. Because of this the patient can accept her help without loss of independence or self-esteem and, therefore, usually shows less resistance. The support is available on the spot, in time of crisis, and can be of the general nonspecific type previously described.

The nurse can stimulate and build up the supportive relationship by giving advice and practical demonstrations of service to the pregnant woman for herself and the infant. Help in preparing the layette, bathing the baby, making the formula, and supervising breast-feeding brings the nurse and the patient into a close collaborative relationship. These procedures should be regarded not only as opportunities for imparting knowledge, but, perhaps more importantly, as occasions for fostering and supporting the ego strength of the mother.

Teaching

Adding to the mother's store of intellectual knowledge increases her ego strength, and this is regarded as a principal mental hygiene function of the nurse. The nurse as a health educator, however, has a difficult job to perform if she wishes to avoid endangering her fundamental wise-sister role. The risk is that she will adopt a teacher role in relation to her patient, and if she does so, her sociological closeness is immediately destroyed. A teacher is typically conceived of by people as having a higher status position than themselves; the nurse who becomes teacher becomes a parent instead of a sister.

An Approach to Community Mental Health

To impart knowledge without assuming teacher status is a technique that has still to be worked out, but it is possible. It is important that the nurse should have a systematic schedule of information to convey, but she should avoid systematic teaching sessions and she should aim at informal teaching techniques – if possible, in group situations, where mothers have an opportunity to teach each other. It is important to stop using the term Mothers' Classes for such groups, and in leading them, the nurse should use democratic methods. She should not set herself up as an expert but rather as someone who is conveying what the experts say. Above all, she should try and help the mothers clarify their own thinking and learn actively rather than receive her teaching passively.

Mobilizing the Environment

This mental hygiene function, which has been described elsewhere in this material, is essentially the province of the nurse.

PROBLEMS AND DIFFICULTIES

My contention that the nurse's closeness to her patient is the fundamental basis for her unique mental hygiene role does not imply that I am opposed to the present efforts of nurses in the United States and elsewhere to raise their professional status to the level of the other specialists in the field. On the contrary, I feel that the difficulties inherent in the interpretation of the patient's needs to the specialists are largely due to their perception of the nurse as a worker of lower status whose reports are not likely to be very valuable. Increasing professionalization, as a result of better preparation, would improve this situation of interdisciplinary collaboration.

In order to act as the bridge and the mediator between the patient and the specialists, the nurse must be regarded by each as being at the same status level as their own group. She therefore has the difficult task of being 'all things to all men'.

The danger at present is that in her efforts to achieve increasing professionalization, she may strive to become a specialist just like all the other specialists, and she may feel that to do so means that she should give up her sibling role with her patients. I can envisage that the idea of growing from a sibling role to a parent role may be a seductive one, but I would warn against 'selling your birthright for a mess of pottage'.

I would emphasize that the concept of the nurse as a wise sister involves a great challenge to nursing education. It implies a higher standard of professional education in order to merit the description 'wise', and this education must be very carefully planned and executed so that the nurse may retain or develop the necessary emotional qualities to allow her to be a sister to her patient. This whole problem merits the most careful consideration by those who shape the policy of the nursing profession.

Techniques of interviewing and handling patients appropriate for the nurse's use need to be studied and developed. At present, most of the techniques in this field have been developed for other disciplines and, unchanged, are not transferable without endangering the nurse's status position. There is also a need to work out how such techniques can be used without increasing the psychological distance between nurse and patient.

A technique which is immediately available for the use of nurses is that of reducing a patient's superficial guilt. An example was given in the case of the expectant woman who had failed in her attempts to terminate her pregnancy. The nurse should be taught how to identify this type of guilt, since it is a potent factor in perverting interpersonal relationships, and she should learn how to deal with the problem as a routine part of her work.

The thinking of the last few years has brought us to the threshold of a great new field in mental health practice, but our basic knowledge in regard to details of the common emotional crises of pregnancy and infancy is still very scanty. We know even less about the special circumstances which are likely to produce mental health hazards. It is surprising how little scientific research has been undertaken to describe the dynamic development of the emotional life of the ordinary pregnant woman.

In order to build up efficient mental health nursing programmes we will have to investigate this area and learn the facts.

For maximum productiveness, such research should be carried out on a collaborative team basis within a framework of all the disciplines, including nursing. This type of multidisciplinary research is difficult to organize and is very costly, but we have reached a stage where it must be regarded as essential.

Examples of the situations which are likely to lead to mental health hazards and should therefore have research priority are : prematurity, Rh negative mothers, illegitimacy, multiple births, failed attempts at abortion, severe illness or death of a near relative during pregnancy, birth trauma in the child, and similar situations. The aim of this research would be to develop specific categories of identifiable circumstances which lead to mental health hazards, and to provide the nurse with indications for specific action in each case.

The mental hygiene work that is based on the nurse's closeness to her patient inevitably involves the nurse herself in emotional problems. The danger is that she will find herself in crisis situations because her own problems are stimulated by those of her patients. This closeness makes her vulnerable in this respect. The likelihood that her patients' problems may set up internal disequilibrium in the nurse is especially great in this field of maternal and child care, because of its significance to every woman, and especially to a woman in the child-bearing years.

One unfortunate result of such a process might be that the nurse might try to work out her own problems through her patients. This might show itself by her usurping the mother's role and becoming possessive of the baby, or by being possessive of the case in relation to the other workers in the field. Another way in which the nurse might attempt to deal with her emotional upset would be by withdrawing from the possibility of involving herself with her patients, either by becoming insensitive to their problems or by increasing her psychological or sociological distance.

It must be emphasized that such emotional upsets are likely to occur in nurses of stable personality if they are doing an efficient mental hygiene job, and must be regarded as a routine occupational hazard.

If this analysis is correct, and our experience indicates that it is, mental hygiene activity by nurses should be planned to include specific safeguards in order to protect the nurse and to minimize her working difficulties.

The best safeguard is an efficient system of technical supervision along the lines which have been worked out in casework and psychotherapy. This is a relatively new idea in nursing; proper methods and organizational framework have still to be developed.

The general nursing supervisor certainly has a part to play. By the atmosphere she creates in her unit, and by the manner in which she conducts herself in relation to the nurses, she sets the tone for their relationship with their patients. She is able to provide a background of nonspecific emotional support which she expresses in her attitude of trust in the capacities of the nurses, her respect for their individuality, and her tolerance for their emotional difficulties. She can also be of limited help in some crisis situations, but her hands are bound by the demands of her leadership role, which forces her to keep the relationship between the nurses and herself on a strictly reality basis. If she permits herself to become involved to any extent in their fantasy life, she will usually experience difficulty in carrying out her tasks as their administrative superior within the agency's hierarchy.

For help in times of emotional crisis, the nurses need someone with whom they can have a freer emotional relationship than is possible with their supervisor – someone outside the administrative hierarchy, with whom they can share their secret emotional reactions without fear of it one day counting against them on the job. This person can allow herself to be involved in their fantasy life since she has no commitments which conflict with this. She can, by her permissiveness, allow the development of the special kind of relationship which can be used to help the nurses achieve a more mature solution of their problems in relation to their work.

I wish to emphasize that this outside supervisor – the mental hygiene consultant – does not carry on psychotherapy with the nurses. She restricts her intervention to helping them overcome the emotional obstacles which prevent them from operating to their maximum efficiency in the case which is brought to consultation. Consultation technique aims at excluding discussion of the private life of the nurse and deals with her problems by helping her find a solution to the patient's difficulties. The benefit to the nurse is obtained vicariously when she is helped to overcome her own troubles, once removed, in her patient.

The mental hygiene consultant nurse is a new arrival and she has much hard work ahead of her in developing her techniques and in establishing her position in the organizational framework of the nursing profession. That she has arrived is a welcome sign of the increasing recognition of some of the important problems I have tried to put before you.

CHAPTER 7

The Role of the Social Worker in the Public Health Setting

I AM going to base what I have to say upon some ideas in preventive psychiatry with which medical social workers are probably already familiar. And, basing myself upon these newer ideas, I am going to try to think aloud about where the present-day social worker may fit in.

I think perhaps the most important idea which governs our thinking in this area is what might be called the ecological theory of emotional health. The evaluation of the state of health or ill-health in an individual can be conceived of as an assessment of a type of internal equilibrium, a balance of intrapsychic forces in a more or less stable state. This is an intrapersonal phenomenon. Significant thinking at the present times ascribes tremendous importance to the concept that what is going on inside that individual is, in the here-and-now situation, part of a complicated interrelated field of forces which includes not only these intrapersonal forces, but also the interpersonal forces between him and the members of his relevant human environment, and between other forces in his wider social environment. The concept is that what is going on inside any individual is in dynamic interplay and is at every moment affected by what is going on outside him. If we wish to get a clear idea of what is happening, we should not divide them.

Another important point is that we are beginning to realize that for too long we have carried over into the preventive field, without very much thinking about it, a basic idea from the field of therapeutic medicine which is not too valuable here, namely, the use of the concept of 'the individual patient' as our reference point. This is a useful focus if we are dealing with an illness which is associated with structural change in an individual. We can isolate this individual with more or less relevance to our investigations and to our treatments. We focus on our patient and then we think of the forces acting upon him, the forces that acted beforehand in order to produce the pathological effect, and the forces that may act afterwards in order to change him either for better or for worse. When we are thinking in preventive terms, this can be a very misleading concept! We are beginning to realize that we should think of a field of forces, of a unit of society – whatever the size of it – rather than of an individual patient.

Another idea which is of importance is the concept of crisis, which is associated, of course, with the idea of equilibrium, because one significant thing about a balance of forces is that sometimes it may get unbalanced. We have discovered that a state of emotional ill-health in an individual is preceded at some time or another in the past by a significant period of disturbance of his previous equilibrium. The person passes through a period of emotional upset which is not in itself an emotional illness, but which leads eventually to a new state which may be the equilibrium of ill-health rather than that of health. Moreover, this crisis, this upset in the internal balance of forces in the individual, is usually precipitated by and is the reaction to a disturbance in the field of forces by which he is surrounded.

In other words, we are thinking of webs of forces with the individual we happen to be looking at as part of them and as reacting to them. The outcome of this crisis, which is usually not too protracted in time, will determine the type of lasting equilibrium which will emerge and whether this is a healthy or an unhealthy state.

Now, what is very important for us to realize is that during this period of crisis, when the balance of forces is unstable, when it is, as it were, 'teetering', a relatively minor force acting for a relatively short time can switch the whole balance over to one side or to the other. If we switch the balance over to one side, we switch it down to the side of an equilibrium which is one of mental health, and if we switch it down to the other side, to one of mental ill-health.

During the particular period of crisis, which may be a few hours or a few days or at most a few weeks, a small force acting for quite a short time produces lasting changes which that force could never produce either beforehand or afterwards. Another point is that, at this moment of crisis, there are certain significant forces in the environment which are especially important, and, of course, outstanding among them is that of the relationship of certain key people to the individual concerned. This relationship may be supportive – that is, tending to weigh the balance down in a healthy direction – or it may be weakening and destructive – that is to say, pushing towards illness.

Even though I talk about how we have to analyse the problem in terms of webs of relationships and how we must avoid the concept of 'the individual patient', I, too, as soon as I begin to discuss it, immediately begin thinking about an individual and the effect of the forces on that individual. At the same time I realize, however, that I have not given the whole story here, and that I have to think also of the other individuals in the field. For instance, there is one experience that all of us who have worked in a child guidance clinic have had. We see a child who comes as the 'patient' with some symptoms for treatment. We enlarge our focus and we find that he has a mother with a disturbed relationship towards him. We think that there is a causal connection. Then we do something to undo this disturbance of relationship between the mother and the child. That is fine, if we are therapeutically oriented, in which case we will say to ourselves, 'Here is my patient, I must cure him.' Perhaps we do cure our patient.

But many of us in the past have been rather rudely surprised to discover that if we followed up such a case and if we widened our focus just a little more, we found that maybe the father, who up to the time of therapy had been reasonably well, now becomes disturbed, or another child, or a grandparent. In other words, the more we narrow our focus, the more we do not need to take into account that our manipulations are causing change in the field as a whole. Of course, we might quite validly say, 'Well, all we're interested in is this particular child'; and yet we may find, if we are honest with ourselves and if we watch the situation afterwards, that we have benefited the child at the expense of the mother or one of the other children. And who knows, and usually we are not in a position to know because we have closed the case, whether the final reaction, even for that child, may not be worse than the first condition?

Now, that leads me on to the question of whether one can adequately analyse any emotional situation. We can. The crucial question is where do we draw the circle of our investigation? We used to draw the circle around the patient, let us say, the child. At that stage all we were interested in was what was going on inside the child, in the intrapersonal difficulties of the child; and we got very proficient in working out techniques of investigation and treatment for these intrapersonal difficulties.

Then we got a bit wiser and we spread the circle of our interest a bit wider, around the mother and the child. We talked about mother-child relationships and their disturbances. And nowadays, I suppose in most places, people are getting a bit restive and they are saying, 'Well, we ought to draw the circle a bit wider still, around the father, the mother, and the child.' And when we do that, we have started on a process and begin to say, 'We ought to take the siblings in, and maybe the grandparents.' We begin to ask ourselves, 'Well, now, what about the father's work situation, what influence does that have?' Then we realize that the child is not always at home, he goes to school. Should we bring the teachers in? And if we bring the teachers into our study, what about the social structure and culture? And if we are going to take that into account, what about the tensions in the surrounding community?

Eventually all these forces from outside narrow down and impinge upon the particular child who was the original patient presented for treatment. And so we can make our analyses in regard to the intrapersonal situation which the person presents, or we can add the interpersonal forces in the small group of the family. We can make a sociological analysis in regard to the structure of that particular community. We can analyse the situation anthropologically from the point of view of the systems of customs and values of that particular culture which sanction certain behaviour of the individuals in that situation and give them the support and protection of the group as a whole.

It now becomes pertinent to ask ourselves, 'Where do social workers come in? What is the role of the social worker in regard to these ideas?' I think that a good way of beginning to think this out is to say that the role of the social worker will obviously be influenced and determined by her previous professional education and experience and by the kinds of skills which she has developed. I think it is clear from my analysis so far that she has got one very obvious role, which is perhaps hardly possible to any other clinical worker, in that she is the specialist in assessing environmental phenomena.

The theoretical concepts that I have referred to offer the social worker new opportunities that she has not had before and, at the same time, a new challenge. This thinking sounds a clarion call to the social worker in the United States to return to her vocation after a period of several years when I feel she has strayed from her traditional path. This she has done when she has altered her focus from the social aspects of casework to the intrapersonal aspects of psychotherapy.

I was recently talking to a visitor from Sweden and he was asking me whether, in the United States, social workers made home visits. I told him, 'Years ago social workers in the U.S.A. did a lot of home visiting. That was when they were interested in the cruder aspects of the environment. And then, as sensitive people, they became aware of certain emotional phenomena, not just of the size of the room or the arrangement of the furniture and the number of people in the family, and so on, but of the emotional factors in the environment. And that's when they came over to start a partnership with the psychiatrists.' I hope I will not be considered presumptuous if I say that in developing this partnership they have been intellectually seduced by psychiatry and its philosophy of the moment.

Until quite recently one found that values among social workers were such that they felt that to do ordinary casework was rather low-quality work. The important thing became to deal with the intrapersonal, emotional factors, to do something which was rather hard to differentiate from the kind of work which psychiatrists call psychotherapy, namely, focusing on the intrapersonal difficulties of the client, handling him in an interview situation, and working out techniques for relieving his intrapsychic conflicts. And I will not say that social workers did better or worse than the psychiatrists from the point of view of results. If I had to train someone *ab initio* as a psychotherapist, I would probably feel that a trained social worker would be a better candidate than a physician.

But I think that the time has now arrived when social workers should realize that they have, in regard to these newer concepts, a tremendous field of opportunity, which is the opportunity to make use of their traditional knowledge of environmental factors, but not in the old way – in a new way which has now been leavened and changed by their increased knowledge of emotional factors and, most important, by their knowledge of the unconscious implications of overt behaviour.

The theme of the unconscious implications of overt behaviour is tremendously important. It is the basis of psychotherapy. But it need not be restricted to psychotherapy, it need not be restricted to the intrapersonal phenomena. Social workers can make use of this knowledge and this sensitivity in regard to the environmental forces which impinge upon people. What, then, are these functions which the social worker might take on in regard to this tremendous field?

First, and this is the very obvious thing, she is *par excellence* the member of a clinical team who can advise where to draw the circle in regard to the strategy of assessing a situation. This is a difficult and important question because we cannot go drawing our circle around the world. There has to be a place where the width of the circle, from the point of view of learning which forces are significant, has to be countered by the width of the circle from the point of view of being able to handle in a practical way the crucial forces. There are certain factors which are going to be critical, and certain which are not. You cannot go into history and economics and politics, and if you did, you would not get anywhere. You might perhaps, at the end of a very long life, get an accurate analysis of a particular situation; but you would not get too far from the practical point of view of doing anything about it.

A clinical team needs someone who is an expert in these environmental factors to say, 'Where do we draw the circle? Do we take in the school in this case? Do we take in the local community tensions in that case? Do we take in the sub-cultural phenomena in the other case? Do we take in the father? The grandmother? Whom do we take into our study?'

And now I come to an important practical point. In order to do this, the social worker must change her habits of work. She must go back bodily into the field. Now maybe some of you started off by spending your time in the field and then worked your way up to being able to have an office with a carpet on the floor. Maybe returning to work in the field may involve the danger of loss of status, as well as undoubtedly being less comfortable!

You can learn something about the field, no doubt, from interviewing the mother and child in your office, but you cannot really learn the essential things you need to know for our present purpose. You cannot learn what are the significant parts to deal with without actually penetrating the environment and getting the information by your sensitivity to the behaviour of the people there. In other words, you will not get the implications of the factors which are operating in the field if you get the information distorted by the eyes and the ears and the unconscious parataxic distortions of someone who is himself emotionally involved in the situation. Most of you have probably discovered by now that if you listen to the story of the wife about her husband you are sometimes very surprised indeed when you go to meet this great big, hulking brute and you find a poor, little drippy sort of chap who would not hurt a fly. It is only by actually penetrating the field that the social worker is going to get the relevant information.

There are techniques to be worked out in regard to assessing the field situation. It is no longer the easy thing that it was twenty years ago, because now you are paying attention not only to the surface manifestations but, in addition, to the deeper implications of those surface manifestations. Possibly one of the reasons why the social workers retired from the field into their offices was because things got too complicated. Once upon a time if you went out on a home visit and someone offered you a cup of coffee, and you wanted to be nice and polite, you took it. Nowadays you have to think, 'Well, what does this mean? She offers me a cup of coffee on this visit but she didn't do this last time. What does it mean that she leaves the door of the room open? What does it mean that she suddenly raises her voice while issuing the invitation? What does it mean that "by chance" she has neighbours visiting her? What does it mean that there's someone there in the corner she doesn't introduce me to?' These used not to be problems. These are now very complicated problems. You have also become sensitive now to what you do. What will happen if you take the coffee? What will it mean to her if you do not take it?

This problem of assessment of the relevant forces in the environment and the role of the social worker in bringing this knowledge into the clinic is linked with another role. And that is that the social worker is by virtue of her skills and her education able to make a unique contribution in regard to the tactical considerations in any case in working out and implementing a plan of preventive intervention. She is usually the only person who can validly say how much of the work in any particular case can be done inside the clinic walls and how much has got to be done out in the field, because she is the only one who really knows the field.

I would now like to turn to techniques of preventive intervention which are appropriate for the social worker. First of all, there are the techniques of direct treatment of interpersonal relationships in the narrower circle, and this is an area where a certain amount of work and research has been done in recent years. Let us take, as our example of such a small unit of society, the family group, which we have now clearly recognized to be an intense field of forces which is highly significant for the mental health of each of its members. A lowering of the general morale of this group or a disturbance of the interpersonal relationships among its members will in many instances eventually lead to emotional illness in one or another of them, and in the children to disorders of personality development.

Now, it is interesting to note that in such situations a psychotherapist can do very little from the practical preventive point of view. Why is this? Let us say that the mother's disordered relationship with her child is in this particular case dependent upon a disorder of her own personality, i.e. an intrapersonal disorder which is manifesting itself by the symptom of a disordered relationship with the child. If we are going to try to prevent the development of neurosis in the child by taking the mother on in psychotherapy, we may succeed; but the expenditure of psychotherapeutic time will be such that our service will be indistinguishable from that of a remedial clinic. I doubt whether the Community Chest gains by paying for adult psychotherapy in place of child therapy! Nor would there ever be hope of community coverage.

But now we know, and this has been shown in France, in Denmark, in the U.S.A., and in Israel, that it is often possible to repair the disorder of interpersonal relationships without having to become involved in taking on that particular person as a psychotherapeutic patient. You can work out techniques which will put the relationship right without your having to become involved in putting the underlying personality problems right at the same time. It is possible for a woman to have a healthy mother-child relationship even if she is neurotic; and it is possible for a woman to have a disturbed mother-child relationship even if her general personality is healthy. We understand this by postulating that the relationship involves only one segment of her personality. Not all her problems are going to focus on the child. Whether

her personality as a whole is neurotic or not, she may attempt to solve only certain of her problems through the child.

Now we can prevent her using the child to solve her problems by means of one of these 'unlinking techniques'. But then we have to ask ourselves, 'In what way is she going to solve these problems?' I suppose one rather good solution, from the community point of view, is that she should solve her problems by developing some stable neurotic symptom. I am not really putting this forward as a practical programme, but let us not forget that neurosis is a community syntonic phenomenon, that is to say, neurosis is the individual's sacrifice for the good of the community. It is not against the community's interests until it reaches a form and a degree where it incapacitates the person to such an extent that he cannot be a reasonable, functioning member of society.

If you think for one moment about the causation of neurosis, you realize that a neurotic symptom represents a solution of a conflict between the individual's interests and the interests of the community. He is solving the conflict at his own expense so that he can say, 'I'm a good member of the community. I will not be aggressive. I will not experience or gratify my instinctual desires. I will bottle them up within me.'

From the point of view of prevention, this is important because what we are worried about is not so much the fact that he is going to solve his conflict on his own person, but that he may solve his problems by manipulating others in his environment, and in this way he may affect many others. One mother with unsolved problems may distort the personality development of five or six children. One teacher or one foreman in a workshop who has some problems unsolved in himself may distort the personality development and the emotional equilibrium of many, many other people who depend on him. This is what we at the Harvard School of Public Health call the 'carrier' of emotional disorder, namely, the key person in a field who is important to many other people and who, when they are in crisis, has the power through his relationship with them to tip them towards health or towards ill-health. He has disordered relationships of such a nature that he acts destructively when other people get into a crisis situation. If you can get hold of such a person, can you do something about him? The answer is, 'You can.'

This whole area has only been opened up in the last few years. The techniques which have been developed have been called by some people 'child-centred treatment of the mother' or 'focused casework'. Other people call it 'segmental treatment'. Call it what you will, it is a technique of interview treatment of a person whereby the worker focuses and delimits the area which is going to be the content of the discussion. This means that he does not allow non-directive, free flow of material.

The worker decides what to let into the interview and what not to let into it. The focus is kept on a narrow segment in regard to the relationships of that key person with the other people – the child, or the other members of the family, or the workers in the factory. How this is done is a matter for study and research. All I wish to say here is that it can be done, and it can be done in certain cases very effectively and very quickly. I am not talking about any kind of 'buttering over' or any kind of 'patting on the back' supportive treatment. I am talking about a radical operation on attitudes and relationships.

The next form of direct intervention, the techniques of which still have to be perfected by the caseworker, is direct help to an individual in crisis. In this, the social worker is operating as a direct, grassroots-level worker. She is present at the moment of crisis. She uses her specific knowledge of the gamut of successful ways of adapting to this crisis and her general knowledge of the way in which people relate to problems and to other people, in order to bring her emotional support quite specifically into this play of forces and to tip the balance down towards a new equilibrium in a healthy direction.

This is a very pointed intervention. In order to succeed we have to know quite a lot about the crisis. We have to know quite a lot about techniques of handling people on such occasions. One important point to bear in mind is that if you press at the right time, you do not have to do it for very long and you do not have to do it very hard. At crisis-time things boil up, and you have an opportunity which you never had before and which you will not have afterwards. The importance of this in regard to community planning is that it gives us the opportunity for expending our skilled work in the most economical way possible at the focal point.

This leads me on to the indirect techniques which social workers may use during crisis. This idea follows, really, from what I have just said. The social worker cannot be present herself during the crisis period of more than a fairly insignificant number of people. But we do know that there are professional workers, representatives of the community, who are normally present during crisis periods. Many of these crises – such as birth, marriage, death, and so forth – are bio-social situations. They have been recognized in a special way in every culture system. Complicated customs, habits, traditions, and folklore have been developed in connection with these periods. What is the purpose of these? They appear to have been designed by the group as a whole to protect and support its individual members.

I think it is fairly certain, and I do not need to say too much about it here, that in a society which is fairly well integrated, that is, where the culture is systematically sustained, there is a minimum of individual emotional breakdown. On the other hand, where a culture has become quite disorganized, for instance among immigrants or transplanted people who have been separated from home, and who, therefore, are just floating from a cultural point of view, with no stability and no external framework or supportive scaffolding, the amount of individual emotional breakdown is phenomenal.

In a stable culture there exist people who are the safeguarding, the caretaking agents of the community, who are normally present at the moment of crisis in order to help individuals on behalf of the community. The biggest problem of preventive psychiatry at the present time is the question of how to help these caretaking people act in an emotionally supportive way during these periods of crisis. The word 'supportive' is somehow rather a feeble word for something which can be so very pointed a weapon against disorder at such times. The important problem is how can we help these caretaking people who are on the spot at the moment of crisis to exert their pressure to tip the balance over to the side of emotional health?

We have done some research at the Harvard School of Public Health on this point and it is one of the main interests in the Community Mental Health Program in Wellesley and in the newly established Mental Health Program in the Whittier Street Public Health Center. We call the techniques which we have been working out in order to solve this problem 'mental health consultation'. The mental health consultant, in this case a social worker, works with the grassroots, caretaking agents of the community with the idea of helping them handle the crises of their clients in their prime. Such caretaking agents have included nurses, teachers, kindergarten teachers, clergymen, public health officers, general physicians, paediatricians, welfare workers, and community leaders.

Early in our work we made a discovery which seemed to us to be highly significant. We found that a caretaking person such as a teacher, who did a very efficient mental hygiene job with most of her pupils, failed completely to handle the problems of a small proportion of them. We found that such a teacher with a class of thirty children would be doing a good job with twenty-five, twenty-six, or twenty-seven of them; but that in the cases in which she failed, she failed at the most important time, namely, when those particular children were passing through crisis periods. She then brought her pressure down on the wrong side of the balance from the point of view of their mental health.

When we examined these cases, we found that the type of child with which any teacher failed, from the point of view of his mental health, was related to certain problems which the teacher had not been able to solve in herself. The teacher's problems, on investigation, might turn out to be primarily intrapsychic or they might very obviously be related to tensions within the school social system or between the school and the community, as for example, in tensions between parents and the teaching staff. Whatever the facts in any individual case, it appeared to be an invariable finding that these forces eventually narrowed down

197

to a disturbance in the relationship between the teacher and the child at that particular time and eventually focused on the child himself. At such moments of crisis the disequilibrium of the child was usually mirrored by a disequilibrium in the teacher. In other words, not only the child, but also the teacher was in a state of crisis. This was usually shown by her losing her professional distance from her pupil and becoming personally, emotionally involved in his situation.

The picture presented by many of these teachers when they complained about the symptoms of one of their pupils resembled very much the familiar picture of the mother complaining of symptoms in her child, which are related to a disturbance in the mother-child relationship. In the same way that such a mother, when talking about her child, can very easily be seen to be referring to her own problems, the story of the teacher in regard to her pupil's difficulties seems to have implications in regard to her own situation.

If the things said at the beginning of this discussion are remembered, such a finding should not be in any way surprising. Both teacher and pupil are reacting in a dynamic way to the web of interpersonal forces of which they are both integral components. The particular child who is complained of at any time is not chosen by chance, but by virtue of the fact that his difficulties at that moment either stimulate or mirror in some way the here-and-now problem of that teacher in the current situation in that school. There are, of course, children with some serious structural disturbance of personality which is relatively uninfluenced by the forces I am talking about. I do not refer to these, but to the much more common situation of a reactive behaviour disorder in a child, which is the usual type for which teachers request advice and help. These are disturbing children but usually not particularly disturbed.

When the teacher is herself in a state of crisis, she is unable to perceive the child as a separate person and is unable to be sensitive to his needs, and is, therefore, not able to help him in his trouble in any adequate way. Instead she reacts to the child's situation in terms of her own problems; and since she herself has been unable to solve these, it is very understandable that what she does in regard to the child is usually not very effective.

In trying to work out methods for dealing with this kind of situation there is one rather obvious fact to bear in mind. The mental health consultant cannot offer psychotherapy to the teacher. If he did so, she would probably kick him out, and quite rightly so. Her private problems are her own business, and it is up to her how she wishes to handle them. She has not defined the consultation situation as one in which her own difficulties are legitimately to be discussed. The consultant, however, has been invited into that situation by the community and has been empowered by that community to interest himself in, and to protect the mental health of, that particular segment of the child population. The community, moreover, implicitly places on the consultant the responsibility to have as wide a range of vision as possible in regard to the factors influencing the child's mental health. The teacher, in so far as she is a loyal community member, accepts the consultant in this role and empowers him to take whatever action is necessary as long as it does not explicitly impinge upon her own personal, private rights. It is in this framework that the technique which we have called 'mental health consultation' has been evolved.

I can describe this technique only briefly here. A preliminary paper has appeared on this subject in the *American Journal of Orthopsychiatry* (1954). This is a paper I wrote jointly with Jona Rosenfeld, a social worker from Israel, on mental health consultation in an organization for immigrant children, in which we described the techniques we had worked out for helping the staff of the residential institutions deal with their problems in regard to handling the children. The technique consists of the consultant entering the child's environment and building up a relationship with the caretaking person, whom we call the consultee. Through the medium of this relationship, he picks up information on two levels. First, on the explicit level, the consultant gets a good deal of information about the details of the disturbance in this particular child and the factors and forces impinging upon him from his environment. At the same time that this explicit information is being gathered, the consultant is constantly sensitive to the under-the-surface implications of the details and manner of telling of the story in regard to the crisis situation of the consultee and of the consultee institution.

These facts can only be picked up by implication and by 'reading between the lines' because the consultee quite likely regards this situation as a professional one into which she should not explicitly intrude her private problems. But since these problems are pressing upon her and since at the moment she is emotionally upset, she cannot help communicating something about them in a non-verbal way. She thinks she is just talking about the child. She is, however, at that moment, in everything she does both in regard to the child and in her relationship with the consultant, talking about the things that are going on inside her. As long as this is only by implication and is not made explicit, the situation is felt by her to be quite safe. One essential point in the mental health consultation technique is that the consultant does not interfere with this defence structure of the consultee and never makes explicit the direct link between the problems of the child and the problems of the caretaking person. Should he do this, he immediately becomes involved in a psychotherapeutic situation which is, as you know, always associated with problems of dealing with resistance. Such problems cannot be dealt with in the fluid situation of a consultation relationship.

The consultant has to pick up the implicit message which is being communicated without interfering with its non-verbal character. He must also learn to reply to this message in a similar, non-verbal way, and his implicit communication must be designed in such a way as to support the emotional strength of the consultee and help tip her balance of forces towards a healthy equilibrium. In this communication, the consultant must accept the defences of the consultee and must not interpret or uncover in an explicit way things which the consultee does not wish at that moment to face.

The consultee does not say, for example, 'I have unsolved problems in my relationship with my mother which are at the moment being stimulated because the headmistress of the school is a motherly person and I am at the moment in conflict with her.' This is much too difficult a problem for her to talk about with a comparative stranger, and it may even be so difficult that she is unwilling to think very clearly about it herself. Instead, she brings up a child for discussion with the consultant and she draws particular attention to the fact that this child is, at the moment, in conflict with his mother. This is very likely no artifact; the child may very well be having troubles with his mother.

But if all the consultant recognizes is that aspect, he is missing the main point of the consultation, namely, why does this consultee at this moment bring this child. A few months later this teacher would probably ask for help with some other child presenting some other problem, and might not feel disturbed about the first child. The reason that she asked for help with this child at this moment is that at this moment this particular problem is important to her. She is disturbed by it; she is in crisis over it.

The way in which such a situation is handled, in this technique, is that the consultant discusses the problem by keeping it centred on the details of the child's difficulties. He discusses the child with a constant awareness of the implications of what he is saying in regard to the consultee's problems. This results in a sort of three-cornered situation, where the consultee and the consultant are discussing the consultee's difficulties under the guise of talking about the child. One of the things which makes this technique so difficult is, however, that the content in regard to the child must be meaningful at that level, and the consultant must constantly be killing two birds with one stone.

I hope that we shall soon have worked out this new technique sufficiently to be able to present it in a systematic way to other workers. It is complicated and difficult, but it is a fascinating technique and certainly it is potentially tremendously important in this field. If it does not turn out to be what we want, then we must find something else that will do the same job. We must work out methods whereby a small number of highly trained people can work with the many caretaking agents of a community who are in so strategic a position during crisis periods to affect the mental health of so large a proportion of the community. If we can succeed in working out some techniques of this nature and if we can get ourselves trained in it, we shall have developed for the very first time a potent instrument whereby we may achieve some kind of approximation of community coverage.

Lastly, a few words about the social worker's responsibilities to the clinic team. I feel that I do not need to say very much on this point. I wish merely to underline two aspects of the social worker's role.

First, I believe that it is the job of the social worker, by virtue of her background and her long and arduous training in dealing with her own emotions in the professional setting, to spread among the other team members a willingness to admit and accept emotional disequilibrium not only in the patients and clients but also among the staff members themselves. Some of us do not realize how very difficult this is for the other people in allied professions to understand because we may have already forgotten how long a time it took us to learn it ourselves, to learn a tolerance of our own humanity.

The second important contribution of the social worker to the team depends upon her knowledge of the supervisory process and of the importance of emotional support for the individual worker at moments of stress. By virtue of this knowledge, the social worker can help the team build up an atmosphere which will be supportive of its individual members, so that when they go out into the field where they will be exposed to all kinds of emotional stresses, they will go out not as individuals, but as emissaries of the group. Teachers in schools of social work must be very familiar with this problem. I believe that social workers have discussed it and dealt with it more effectively than psychiatrists, and by now must have amassed a considerable body of knowledge which might be made available.

These are among the most valuable contributions which a social worker may make in a clinical team. The social workers and I have managed to make some reasonable contribution along these lines in our Family Health Clinic at Harvard. We did not manage this entirely without difficulty both for ourselves and for our colleagues. People may after all be very competent in their practice of the allied professions without having learned how to be comfortable about their own personal emotional involvement in a professional problem. It was not surprising that some of our colleagues were, in the beginning, rather ashamed to say, 'Oh, I hate this patient. She really gets in my hair.' Nowadays they are beginning to be able to say such things and to feel confident that they will not be rejected by the other people on the team, but on the contrary, supported in their efforts to disentangle their own emotional upset from the presenting professional problem. It is a source of great relief to an individual team member to know that the group will help him to avoid transferring to his relationship with his client his own disequilibrium of the moment.

This certainly does not mean that I am suggesting that the social worker treat psychotherapeutically the problems of her fellow team members. It does, however, mean that she says to them, in effect, 'You are entitled to have your emotional problems, and I have them too. We all have them, but they need not necessarily interfere with our work. As long as we stand together, we can have our personal problems and still do a good job. In any case, we cannot and need not deny that we, too, have emotions which may be disturbed, since this is after all one of the essential attributes of our common humanity.'

In conclusion, I should like to underline something which has been implicit in all I have tried to say. The consideration of this topic of the role of the social worker in preventive psychiatry, at present, throws up many questions and very few definite answers; but some of the questions and some of the attempts at answers point to fascinating and challenging new vistas. For the first time we have glimpses of attainable, practical goals, but it is clearer than ever before that much hard research lies ahead. In this exciting work the social worker has an honourable and a difficult part.

REFERENCE

Caplan, Gerald, & Rosenfeld, Jona (1954). 'Techniques of Staff Consultation in an Immigrant Children's Organization in Israel.' *Amer. J. Orthopsychiat.* **24**, 42–62.

CHAPTER 8

The Role of the Family Doctor in the
Prevention of Emotional Disorder

THE aetiology of emotional disorder in any individual case is very complicated. Many interacting factors are involved, including those based on constitution, childhood experiences, later life problems and their solution, and details of the unfolding of the processes of growth and development in interaction with the forces of the emotional and material environment.

If one looks at this problem from an epidemiological point of view it is still complicated, but it is simpler: by this I mean a study of the factors in one community which are responsible for its having a higher incidence of cases of emotional disorder than another community. Such studies isolate certain common factors which operate to influence all members of a community. These factors do not determine the fate in any individual case, but they lead to community-wide differences in the frequency of certain psychological illnesses.

Viewed from this standpoint it is possible to discover certain general factors which can be combated on a community-wide level. Programmes to alter these factors may not affect the fate of any particular person but are likely to reduce the number of cases which occur during a subsequent period in that community.

In connection with these factors the following consideration seems important: the mental health of an individual is dependent on the continuous satisfaction of special requisites in the patterns of his psychological interaction with certain other people. We can speak loosely about a person having psychological needs which have to be satisfied in his interactions with others. The most obvious need is the basic psychological stimulation of having people to talk to. For years we have realized that isolation has a potent harmful effect on mental health. For centuries men have tortured their fellows by marooning them on desert islands, by solitary confinement in prisons, or by ostracism in the social setting. The list of needs also includes the opportunity to give and receive love and affection, to be dependent and to be depended on, to satisfy cravings to be controlled and to control, and to be a member of a social group in which one's identity and personality are respected and accepted, so that one's achievements are rewarded by praise and one's difficulties are lightened by sympathy and understanding.

In all cultures there exist within the structure of the society small groups of people who are bound together by significant emotional ties, and within these groups the psychological needs of the individual members are satisfied. Biological ties are usually the basis of these fundamental groupings, and some form of family structure is universal. In different cultures the pattern of families varies, but, whether we study the small family of modern Western urban culture, the large extended family of earlier Western rural culture or certain present-day Oriental cultures, or the matriarchal families of other cultures, we find that certain roles or tasks of psychological significance are allotted by tradition to each of the family members, that the sum of these tasks usually satisfies the needs of all the members, and that this sum is distributed among the members of the group so that no necessary role is left out.

In recent years we have discovered that the interactive possibilities afforded by the intact structure of the family are as necessary to mental health as the provision of adequate nutritional supplies is to physical health. When the traditional pattern of any family is altered by situational factors, the mental health of its members is endangered. This danger is greatest for the younger children, in the same way that nutritional deficiencies are most dangerous during early developmental phases, but the danger is also present for the mature adults.

Another similiarity to physical nutrition is that if all goes well we do not usually realize the importance of these factors. The satisfaction of needs in an intact family takes place silently and automatically. It is only when the family structure is deficient that difficulties become obvious; since families are ubiquitous, it has taken us a long time to realize the obvious fact of their importance for mental health and the close connection between defects in their structure and subsequent emotional disorders among certain of their members.

IMPORTANCE OF THE FAMILY PHYSICIAN IN PROMOTING MENTAL HEALTH

From all this it follows that professional workers who deal with people as members of a family have a special place in programmes of mental health promotion. The family physician is a worker with a uniquely important role in this regard. He is usually called in to a family to handle symptoms of physical disorder in one or more of its members. In dealing with this traditional task he may well add another dimension to his practice and focus his interest on those elements of the situation which involve dangers to the social structure of the family group, therefore involving dangers to the future mental health of its members. The concept of the family as a unit, and the physician as a worker with responsibilities to the whole unit, implies not only that he may accept as a patient any individual family member but also that when he is called in to deal with the symptoms of one member he will widen the focus of his interest to include all the others, whether from the point of view of their involvement in the aetiology of his patient's condition or from the point of view of the effects of his patient on them as a group. This responsibility has been clear for years in cases of contagious disease, but we now realize that it applies equally, if not more so, to the social and psychological side-effects and sequelae of any illness. This latest insight is, as is often the case in medicine, a reformulation of old traditional knowledge; the family physicians in our parents' generation understood this quite well, although they may not have been able to spell it out as explicitly as we can nowadays. Increasing complexity in the medical sciences, increasing specialization, and increasing concentration on the exciting new discoveries in somatic medicine have to some extent pushed these old insights into the back of our minds. In the hurly-burly of busy practices, and in the absence of strong protagonists, they have fallen into disuse.

Moreover, the former training of physicians by the apprentice system allowed young men to acquire many of the skills of psychosocial management of the family by modelling themselves on the practice of experienced preceptors. The knowledge they acquired was not to be found in books but in the life situations of their apprenticeship. Nowadays the old type of apprenticeship is usually missing, and the books still say very little about all this – at least very little that is useful at a practical level – because the writers of these books have usually not carried out their studies within the framework of the actual situations of general medical practice but in the very specialized and unique conditions of psychiatric clinics and psychological laboratories.

Exhortations by psychiatrists that the family physician should play his part in promoting mental health are no great help. The family physician asks, 'Exactly how should I do this?' and the psychiatrist usually has no concrete answer. In what follows I shall attempt to begin to give a concrete answer – or at least to indicate specific avenues for practical exploration.

Before ending this introduction, I should like to mention one other point which supports the importance of the family physician in community programmes of preventive psychiatry. He is one of the key community workers who have contact with people when they are in a state of crisis. Physical illness may be a turning-point which determines a change in the whole course of a person's existence; it is important to realize that during the relatively short period of the few weeks or months of the illness all kinds of decisions may be made, and all kinds of psychological reorientations, as well as alterations in the structure and functioning of families, may be worked out which will affect the type of interpersonal relationships and character of intrapersonal functioning for a long time to come.

Psychiatrists have recently joined the ranks of those who are very interested in the way people solve the emotional and social problems of periods of life crisis. Previously, it was mainly novelists and dramatists who were interested in this topic, but nowadays we psychiatrists realize that the future mental health of people may be determined at crisis times by the quality of their problem-solving methods. One type of solution of a set of problems may lead to greater mental health, which explains why many people become more mature as a result of satisfactorily overcoming life's difficulties. Another type of solution may lead to mental ill-health, either immediately or in the future, and either directly for that individual or indirectly for his dependents owing to damage of his emotional relationships with them.

People become emotionally disturbed during these crisis periods, but the anxiety, depression, tension, and hostility are not to be confused with symptoms of psychiatric illness, which they superficially resemble. They are the signs in the emotional sphere which show that an active struggle is in process inside that individual in his attempts to wrestle with his problems. At the end of the few weeks of crisis these symptoms will disappear, once some kind of solution has been achieved. This solution may be a healthy one. On the other hand it may be an unhealthy one, and in that case either at once or in the future the individual will manifest neurotic or psychotic symptoms which represent a pathological way of dealing with his life problems through some form of irrational and psychologically distorted pseudo-solution.

The most important point for preventive psychiatry is that the type of problem-solving during a crisis can be powerfully influenced by the helpful or hindering intervention of other people, both in the family circle and from the outside, in the form of the physician and other community agents. When the balance of forces is upset in a crisis a minimal intervention may produce major and stable results by determining on which side the balance will come down.

This means that the operations of the family physician during any of his visits for whatever reason to a family in crisis may have a major effect on the pattern of resolution of that crisis and on the members' future mental health.

I wish now to concentrate on examples of certain practical implications for the operations of the family physician that arise out of these theoretical considerations.

SAFEGUARDING THE INTEGRITY OF FAMILY STRUCTURE

The general practitioner has many opportunities in his practice to help keep families from breaking up temporarily or permanently; or, if this cannot be avoided, to help them find substitutes for roles which the family break-up has left vacant.

Most important is the prevention of separation of the mother from the family circle or from one of her children. Bowlby (1951) and other workers have shown fairly conclusively that the separation, for any appreciable time, of the stable mother figure from a child during the first few years of its life exerts a damaging effect on the development of the child's personality, leading in severe cases to extreme forms of psychological and psychosomatic illness. If the physician is aware of this, he will be alert to explore practical alternatives to any plan for removing a mother or a child from the home because of illness. Often the removal from home is quite inevitable because the nature of the illness demands hospitalization, but frequently the physician may be able to plan for this absence to be short and for the remainder of the treatment to be carried out at home. The fact that the mother is physically incapacitated certainly will influence her ability to fulfil many of the demands of the mother role, but her mere presence in the home will allow her, through repeated contacts with other family members, to maintain the emotional bonds of comfort and sympathy and mother love which are the emotional nutrients the others need.

Of course such a plan implies the need for nursing and home-maker [home-help] services to care for the patient at home and to take over her housewifely duties. The physician should be active in helping the family secure such services either from the ranks of the extended family of grandparents, aunts, sisters, and cousins; from neighbours and friends; or, if these are not available, from professional workers. When the latter are not available I believe that local physicians should actively campaign among appropriate community agencies for their provision. Family physicians should be as interested in the adequacy of community agency provision in this area of homemaker services as they are in the standards of their local hospitals, since both affect the quality of the professional care they can give their patients.

The feeling in regard to hospitalization of young children should be that of avoiding or postponing or shortening it whenever possible. With modern methods of diagnosis and treatment and effective home nursing, many types of cases which in the past necessitated admission to children's hospitals can be treated at home.

When separation is inevitable the physician should encourage frequent and regular visiting to maintain channels of communication and continuation of the emotional links.

In 1952 in England, as a result of Bowlby's researches, the Ministry of Health issued a directive to permit and encourage daily visiting in children's wards. In the United States this is also becoming common paediatric practice, and some new children's hospitals have facilities for parents to sleep in the ward near their child and help with certain nursing procedures. This has led to inevitable complications in ward management and new problems for the nursing staff, but none of these has proved insoluble and they are a small price to pay for the results in terms of safeguarding the personality development of the children.

The physician interested in the whole family should also be on the alert for the neglect of the other children when one child is hospitalized. He should try to mobilize the efforts of other family members to cover the hiatus left when a mother is concentrating her efforts on the ill child, and his activity in this regard should not stop when the ill child comes home. We are familiar with many cases of neurotic disturbance in children which started during periods of parental neglect owing to the illness of a sibling.

If the mother has to go into the hospital, the physician should try to promote communication from her to the other family members, particularly the children, through frequent verbal and written personal messages; he should also use his best efforts to help the rest of the family stay together in their home. If the family stays together they may close their ranks and take over, as a group, some of the absent member's functions, whereas if they are split up this group strength is dissipated.

In order to keep the family together the physician may have to mobilize other family members to come in and do the house-keeping, or he may have to call in a homemaker. Placing the children as individuals in other homes may seem the easier way, but it is actually more expensive in both the short run and the long run.

Another area where the family doctor can give invaluable mental health help is that of helping the father take over some of the maternal role left vacant by the absence of his wife. Husbands may need support and explicit encouragement and advice in mothering their children during this period and in assuming unaccustomed leadership in housekeeping. Some men may be rather inhibited in doing what is needed because of false feelings of shame about such activities being effeminate. The physician can watch out for this and throw the power of his prestige behind the medical prescriptions to the hesitant father.

When the separation of the mother is permanent owing to death or desertion the physician should interest himself actively in helping the family plan for her replacement by a substitute. Assistance in this direction, as in the other issues which have been mentioned, may be obtained from a family social agency; but the family physician, who is the professional person with continuing contact and responsibility for the whole family, should help in mobilizing this assistance and should co-ordinate these activities with his own and with those of other helping agents such as clergymen and teachers.

The Family Doctor in the Prevention of Emotional Disorder

The physician should be equally active if it is the father and not the mother who is separated from the family by illness, death, or social factors, such as employment demands or wartime needs. A wife needs her husband's support, and children need the controlling influence of a father-figure. This issue has been relatively neglected until recently. Interest in it has now been aroused by the realization that many common disorders of personality development in children, which lead to delinquency, have been influenced by the absence of a stable controlling father during the child's upbringing, so that the external discipline which is the precursor of the internal discipline of the socialized person has been missing or defective.

If there is no man in the house, the role of discipliner of the children devolves largely on the mother, and she may need the support of the physician, himself a potent father-figure, in order to add this to her other roles. It may also be possible for him to help her out directly in certain crisis situations and to invoke the help of teachers and recreational group leaders.

Perhaps by now it seems that I am advocating turning the general practitioner into a social worker. Nothing is further from my intention. His primary role must remain that of the practitioner of the healing arts; but if our talk of treating the whole person rather than the diseased organ is to be more than a mere slogan, we must expect the physician to add an interest in some of the above psychosocial points to his traditional preoccupation with physical functioning. The family physician may well realize that his role in the family provides him with both the responsibility and the opportunity to affect its functioning in ways which will have direct effects on the health of its members. So long as mental health and mental illness were conceived of as being quite separate from physical health and physical illness, the physician could afford to neglect some of these issues; but nowadays such a dichotomy is hard for most of us to accept and very hard indeed for the general practitioner who deals not with bits of people or special aspects of their functioning, as isolated in special clinics, but with the whole fabric of life within the family circle in the home.

SAFEGUARDING HEALTHY RELATIONSHIPS

The satisfaction of individual psychological needs in the family is dependent not only on the preservation of the integrity of its structure but also on the quality of the enduring interpersonal relationships among its members. The mother may not be geographically separated from her child, for example, but her prevailing feelings toward him may be so anxious, ambivalent, or rejecting, that she cannot perceive his needs, or, if she does, she may have no interest in satisfying them.

Once disordered relationships between family members have fully developed, treatment by a psychiatric specialist is usually needed to improve them; unless such intervention is forthcoming, a significant proportion of the people will eventually need psychotherapy for manifest psychiatric illness. In the past few years, however, we have discovered that the disordered relationships which are harmful take quite a time to develop to their full pathogenic intensity and that during this period the family physician may interrupt this harmful development. His helpful intervention can best be focused at certain crucial periods when disorders in relationships are most apt to occur in response to characteristic temporary situational factors.

Pregnancy. One such crucial period, both for the development of the mother-child relationship and for the other interpersonal relationships in the family, is the period of pregnancy. The mother's relationship with her new baby does not begin at his birth but is being built up during her pregnancy; the complicated metabolic development of this period has a characteristic effect on her emotional functioning, which in turn has reverberations on the emotional life of the family as a whole. These reverberations may lead to changes in the way the family members relate to the expectant mother and to each other, and these changes may become stable and may have far-reaching consequences for mental health by altering the pattern of need satisfaction within the family circle.

Recent studies (Caplan, 1957, 1959) on the emotional manifestations of normal pregnancy have yielded information about characteristic series of emotional changes which occur in many expectant mothers and which are apt to frighten them and to interfere with family life. The physician who knows the details of this predictable development may make powerful use of this knowledge.

His main technique will be anticipatory guidance, whereby he warns the patient and her husband ahead of time what to expect and thus gives them the chance of preparing themselves psychologically for the difficulties. For instance, quite early in pregnancy the physician should have a joint interview with husband and wife and let them both know that many women become more irritable and more sensitive than usual during pregnancy because of the complicated and little-understood somatopsychic factors; therefore, if in this case the expectant mother suddenly gets angry with minor provocation, laughs or weeps for no adequate reason, or has sudden attacks of depression, neither she nor her husband need get alarmed. These changes, however, dramatic, are not preliminary signs of psychiatric illness and they will disappear after delivery.

At this early conference the physician will also be well advised to mention the likelihood of changes in the pregnant woman's sexual desire and performance. Changes in appetite are frequent in pregnancy, and this relates not only to foods but to sex. In regard to this topic the physician not only gives needed anticipatory guidance but often is able to act as a channel of communication between husband and wife in relation to topics which in our culture may not be easily discussed between them. In the absence of necessary knowledge and in the presence of communication blocks so that difficulties cannot be worked out by discussion, tensions may easily arise between husband and wife, based on distorted interpretations of each other's attitudes. A wife, not infrequently, gets very upset if she loses her sexual desire or capacity for orgasm; she imagines she has become permanently frigid or that she is losing her love for her husband and that he will reciprocate in kind. A husband sometimes fears that his wife is rejecting him because he made her pregnant, and sometimes he seeks alternative sources of sexual satisfaction as a reaction to this imagined rejection. Such unfortunate fantasies can be easily alleviated by the physician's prior discussion of the realities of the situation. He can also help both parties become aware of the strain under which each will be labouring during pregnancy and help them pay special attention to the need to support and sympathize with the partner's difficulties and to make allowances for signs of tension.

Such joint interviews with husband and wife, which should if possible be repeated at least once or twice more during the pregnancy, have a more essential function than just the smoothing out of expected difficulties in the marital relationship, important as this is. My studies have shown that toward the middle of pregnancy most women become more passive and demanding of affection than usual. Instead of being the giving person in the home, actively attending to the needs of others, they now turn in on themselves and feel the need to sit around and be waited on. My studies have also shown that the adequate satisfaction of these needs for increased attention and affection not only is important for increasing the expectant mother's comfort but also plays an important part in preparing her for adequate motherhood in the first few months after delivery. If she receives enough affection during pregnancy, she can give out enough affection to the baby. Those women who are deprived during pregnancy later have a tendency to deprive their babies.

Recognition of this by the physician allows him to play an important role in ensuring adequate emotional supplies at the crucial early period of the newborn infant's life. He cannot give the expectant mother affection himself, but he can try to make sure she gets it from the natural sources. There are many cultural and psychological factors which may block a husband's demonstrations of affection during pregnancy. He may be so irritated by his wife's petulant behaviour and by her inability to afford him his usual sexual satisfaction that he turns away from her. He may be frightened by her increased demands, and he may feel she is changing her personality and becoming lazy and spoiled. He may resent what he feels is her exploitation of the privileges of pregnancy. His feelings of security in his manly role, which are in our culture often weakened by the lack of respect we pay to expectant fathers, may be further endangered by his wife's demands that he take over some of her maternal functions in the work in the house or caring for the other children.

The physician has the opportunity during his joint conferences with husband and wife, or if necessary during an individual interview with the husband, to prevent the difficulties which may emerge from these factors. He can reassure the husband as to the normality of his wife's reactions and as to their temporary nature, and he can enlist the husband's active help in preparing for the baby by, as it were, 'charging up his wife's battery of affection', so that she can eventually pass the emotional supplies on to the baby. Most important, the physician can by his own attitudes during these meetings help increase the husband's feeling of respect for the importance of his own role as an expectant father. This may help to prevent a not infrequent cause of family difficulty after the baby arrives, when some fathers are hampered in their paternal role by feelings of jealousy in regard to the baby.

I do not wish to leave this very brief reference to the physician's preventive role in emotional disorders originating during pregnancy without mentioning the results of some recent research which has specific practical implications. My studies have shown that certain traumatic events occurring during the period of pregnancy exert a powerful harmful effect on the future mother-child relationship. Such events include the severe illness or death of a near relative of the expectant mother, particularly of a parent, her husband, or one of her children. It is very easy for the woman to displace some of her painful feelings about such an event to her relationship with her unborn child, and her attitudes toward him get distorted by irrational ideas, such as identifying him as a reborn representative of the dead person or blaming him and sacrificing him because of unresolved feelings of personal guilt in connection with the bereavement. The physician should be especially on guard to ensure an adequate process of mourning along lines I shall describe below, and he should help the mother to see and to feel that her new baby is an individual in his own right and has to be recognized and treated as a person with a quite separate fate from everyone else, including the dead person.

Abortion. Another traumatic event during pregnancy which is likely to have a major harmful effect on the future mother-child relationship is an attempt by the mother to abort herself, if this act is against the rules of her culture and traditions, and especially if she keeps it as a guilty secret. It is this guilt which blossoms in secret fantasies and which invades and distorts the relationship with the child. If nothing is done about it, the chances are high that a particularly pernicious disorder of the child's personality will eventually be produced. The important point is that this pathological sequence of events can usually be easily interrupted by the family physician, if he identifies either during pregnancy or soon afterwards what has happened. The technique to be used is one which is not usually a part of the general practitioner's therapeutic armamentarium but one which can be fairly easily learned, namely, specific reduction of conscious guilt. I have discussed this at some length in a recent paper (Caplan, 1954), and here I will only mention it briefly. It consists essentially of the physician helping the woman to talk about what she has done in two or three short interviews, in which he adopts an understanding and nonjudgemental attitude toward her behaviour, without in any way pretending that what she did was a good thing and yet with the clear demonstration that despite what she has done he continues to accept her as a worthwhile person.

DIRECT HELP TO PEOPLE IN CRISIS

The traditional role of the physician brings him into contact with many people during the critical period when they are wrestling with acute life problems, and at such times he can exert a particularly powerful effect on their mental health by steering them toward adequate solutions and away from maladaptive solutions. The clearest example of this is in connection with problems of bereavement.

Bereavement

Eric Lindemann (1944), my colleague at Harvard, has carried out some interesting studies on the nature of the process of mourning which carry clear and specific implications for medical practice. He has found that a bereaved person goes through a well-defined process in adapting to the death of the relative, that this process usually takes four to six weeks to complete, and that it is characterized by a succession of specific psychological steps with accompanying emotional side-effects. It seems that when a key figure is removed by death or desertion from a person's life, that person has to work quite hard, psychologically, in order to adapt to the loss and in order to fill in the resulting emotional hiatus.

Lindemann also found that whereas the majority of people manifest these characteristic mourning reactions, which show they are satisfactorily doing their 'grief work', and recover their psychological and psychosomatic equilibrium by the end of the four to six weeks, a small but significant group of bereaved people do not show these changes, or show them in distorted form; many of these people either immediately or later show definite and sometimes extreme signs of psychiatric or psychosomatic illness, particularly depression and disorders of the gastro-intestinal tract, such as peptic ulcer or ulcerative colitis.

Lindemann postulates a direct causative link between the absence of a normal mourning process and the later development of these illnesses. He has also shown that sometimes these illnesses can be interrupted by helping the patients revive the problems of their bereavement and belatedly do their undone grief work.

Among the characteristic manifestations of a healthy mourning reaction are withdrawal of interest from the affairs of daily life and business, feelings of mental pain and loneliness, weeping, disorders of respiratory rhythm with frequently repeated deep sighs, insomnia, loss of appetite, and – most characteristic – preoccupation with the image of the deceased person, usually in connection with the revival of numerous memories of joint activities with him. Lindemann feels that this last phenomenon is the key to understanding the essence of the mourning process. The bereaved person withdraws his energy from most of the aspects of everyday life and concentrates it on reviewing, detail by detail, those aspects of his past life which were enriched by his association with the deceased. In each of these life segments he has to realize afresh the pain of his loss and rather concretely to experience its permanence. In each of these segments he has to make a special act of resignation to the inevitable. This can only be achieved through suffering, but not until it is completed can the person achieve mastery and independence in that segment of his life, so that he can return to normal activity and emotional stability.

Each bereaved person must do this grief work for himself, and mourning is a lonely process; but the traditions of most cultures illustrate to us that neighbours and friends and representatives of the larger community can help the mourner both by the general emotional support of condolence and by practices which permit him or encourage him to go through the steps of his grief work. In our modern culture the weakening of religious and other cultural systems of values and traditions has thrown many people largely on their own emotional resources, and the family physician is one of the people whose work may call them to step into the breach. In doing so in this area he may well try to enlist the support of the priest or clergyman or rabbi, each of whom has his own traditional approach to these problems.

In order to understand specifically what the family physician might do to help the bereaved person mourn successfully, it is helpful to list some of Lindemann's findings among the unsuccessful mourners, who later developed various illnesses. No single simple picture was characteristic of this group, but combinations of the following reactions were common. Instead of withdrawing interest from daily life many of them showed more business activity than usual and by diverting their interest to the problems of outside life appeared to escape the inner turmoil of mourning. They did not weep. They felt little or no pain, either saying they felt numb and empty or showing a strange cheerfulness. Many of them showed marked hostility, often directed toward the physicians and nurses who had cared for the deceased. In all cases there was an absence of preoccupation with the deceased, and on direct questioning many said they were quite incapable of recalling in memory the image of the deceased person. The overall picture which was most commonly found was an attempt to deny the emotional importance of the whole business and to get on with problems of living without the burden of mourning. In the short run the external emotional manifestations of this group seemed easier and happier than the group of active mourners, but in the long run many of them paid very dearly for their temporary ease.

The guideline for the physician who wishes to profit from these studies is to try and help his patients grieve along the lines of the first group and to be particularly active in giving his help whenever he recognizes in one of his patients, during the mourning period, signs which resemble those of the maladaptive group. Experience has shown that to help such people grieve successfully it is not necessary to know the inner psychological reasons for their being hampered in this regard. The uncovering of these deeper complications is not necessary; all that seems important is to get them by whatever means to dwell on the image of the deceased and to go over and over in their minds the many activities which they shared with him in the past, in order little by little to realize that from now on he will be missing from their lives. What is also necessary is for the physician to give the patient the full measure of his emotional support and sympathy in bearing the pain of this process and for him to mobilize other sources of support within the family and outside it. In this regard the physician should realize that emotional support depends, among other factors, on the quantity of personal interaction, so he should realize the special importance of even short extra visits to his patient during the mourning period, or, if these are not possible under the pressures of a busy practice, at least of phone communication. Since the pathological sequelae of inadequate mourning are usually so severe, these extra visits are well worth while.

When the physician is not able on his own to stimulate a

proper mourning reaction, when his efforts to enlist the aid of ministers of religion and members of the extended family also lead nowhere, and when mourning is absent or continues without apparent resolution long after the expected period of four to six weeks, the physician would be well advised to take active steps to refer the patient to a psychiatrist at that stage and not wait for the psychiatric illness to develop. This is a situation where a specialized 'stitch in time' may well 'save nine'.

Other Crises

Space does not permit me to go into detail about other examples of direct help by the physician to people in crisis, and I hope that some general principles may have emerged from my discussion of help with bereavement. I wish, however, to make brief supplementary mention of two other crises commonly met in medical practice, the crisis faced by parents who have to adapt to the realization that their baby has a congenital abnormality or is mentally defective, and the crisis of a patient or his relatives having to adapt to a chronic or an incurable illness, a major disability, or to death itself. These situations all call for special activity on the part of the physician, in addition to the customary 'frank' or 'not so frank' talk.

The physician must face the fact that the impact of the news of the diagnosis is likely to be followed by a period of psychological reorientation similar to the grief work of the mourning period and interestingly enough also lasting for about four to six weeks. Patients and their relatives should not be expected to handle these psychological burdens on their own. They may need a good deal of support from the physician in facing the painful implications of the situation and help in avoiding facile escape into denial or obliteration of the problem by wish-fulfilling fantasies. The physician should try to help them keep the problem in consciousness during this period and deal with its implications piece by piece. It is remarkable the power that ordinary people have to adapt to reality, however unpleasant. It is not realities but dreams which 'make cowards of us all', and in so far as the problem is allowed to sink into dreams and into fantasies it gets removed from the strength which derives naturally from our universal adaptive mechanisms.

On the other hand, the physician should realize that in its initial impact a problem may be quite overpowering and some partial or initial denial is a fundamental defence mechanism. He should not interfere with this, nor with the occasional rest periods during the adaptation process when the patient tries for a while to forget his problems by diverting his interest to other matters. In fact, the physician who knows his patient may be able to recognize when he is becoming too fatigued by facing the unfaceable, and he may then prescribe a temporary respite by diversion or drugs. He should be on the alert, however, to call a return to the fray once the rest period has resulted in the replenishment of resources.

I should like to sound here a word of warning against the indiscriminate and continuous use of tranquillizing drugs for people in crisis. Studies are at present under way to determine not only their pharmacophysical ill-effects but also their possible psychological complications; among the latter I predict we shall probably find that, by damping down too drastically the impact of crisis situations, tranquillizers may be preventing the active processes of healthy adaptation to important life difficulties and thus laying the stage for subsequent psychiatric illness.

NEED FOR PSYCHIATRIC CONSULTATION

The family physician who seriously wishes to enlarge the scope of his practical operations in order to cater to the mental health needs of his patients and their families would be well advised to build up a collaborative working relationship with a psychiatrist of his choice. If a psychiatrist is not available, such help can also be obtained from a well-trained clinical psychologist or a psychiatric social worker. The important thing is wherever possible to use the same person each time, so that the two can learn each other's language and ways of working.

In talking about consultation I do not have in mind the occasional necessity to refer a patient with some psychiatric illness to

An Approach to Community Mental Health

a specialist for investigation and treatment. This will certainly be necessary, and the more sophisticated the family physician becomes in dealing with emotional problems in his patients the earlier he will be able to identify such conditions and the more easily and surely he will be able to effect the referral procedure.

More Effective Understanding and Management

The kind of consultation I am particularly referring to here is different: it is consultation by the general physician with the psychiatric specialist in order to enlist the latter's help in rendering the family physician's own understanding of the case and his own management of it more effective. However well trained the general physician may be, he will inevitably come across situations involving the emotional life of his patients which are outside the area of his previous learning and experience. The psychiatrist may, by discussing the case with him, be able to enlarge his understanding and to deepen his insight by pointing to the relevance of certain items of information about the field of forces which the physician had previously ignored. The psychiatrist's specialized knowledge of patterns of intrapsychic functioning and unconscious motivation may allow him to explain previously puzzling aspects of the patient's personality and those of his relatives which throw new light on their behaviour and afford new opportunities for helpful action by the physician. It is very important for the doctor to tailor his intervention in the family to the special individual personality characteristics of its members. Most family physicians will build up a store of relevant knowledge of the weaknesses and strengths of their patients from their years of experience with them, but every now and again there will be some reactions which are quite unexpected and the physician may find his best efforts frustrated. On such occasions the psychiatrist's knowledge of the deeper unconscious aspects of personality functioning may clarify the situation so that the physician may find a new way to help his patient.

Improving Use of the Self

Another type of help which the physician may expect from the mental health consultation is that of sharpening and improving his own use of the self in his professional medical functioning. A physician constantly makes use of different aspects of his personal influence on his patients as part and parcel of his daily work. This use of the effect of one human being who is being helpful on another who is in need becomes especially important in dealing with those needs which are predominantly emotional rather than physical.

Unfortunately, although physicians make use of personal influence all the time in their medical practice, this usually remains an amateur, somewhat haphazard set of operations with most physicians rather than a consciously directed professional therapeutic instrument. Some physicians have a more consistently therapeutic personal effect on patients than others, and we ascribe this to innate personality gifts or to a generalized 'bedside manner' of uncertain origin. Even these physicians often fail in their efforts to support or stimulate or reassure certain patients, and when they fail they can no more understand why this has happened and deal with the consequences than they can understand their successful cases. The average physician is no better off when it comes to understanding his own special emotional reactions to certain patients – his feelings of liking and warm protectiveness, his irritability and anger, his frustration, his anxiety, or sometimes his guilty withdrawal. He does his best to control these feelings and not allow them to interfere with his objective medical approach, and his training usually helps him to succeed – but often at the expense of becoming rather distant and cold. It is the rare general physician who is able to capitalize consciously, both for diagnostic and for therapeutic purposes, on his awareness of his own feelings as they are stimulated by the behaviour of his patient.

The psychiatrist, on the other hand, has by a long and arduous training not only learned to know and accept his own human reactions in his reciprocal interaction with his patients but he has learned to make explicit and differentiated use of them in the professional setting. Through the consultation process the physician may gain from him some understanding and skill in this matter. This will only come gradually, which is another reason for working with the same consultant over a lengthy period. This is not a matter of the giving or the receiving of intellectual prescriptions but the emotional education which comes from numerous discussions about the details of practical life situations and one's feelings about them.

Consultation, a Two-way Process

So far I have talked as though the psychiatrist were the teacher and the family physician the pupil in the consultations, and to some extent this is so; but the physician who imagines that all he will have to do is to ask questions and get the answers from the psychiatrist will be sadly disappointed. He will quickly discover that with all his specialized knowledge the psychiatrist does not have many answers to the circumscribed questions about the practical issues of management of ordinary patients in the situation of general practice.

I said before that mental health consultation is a joint collaborative endeavour, and what I meant to imply is that it has to be a two-way process, in which not only the psychiatrist but also the physician must be an active partner. It is essential for the physician to realize that he must take active steps to educate the psychiatrist during these consultations so that he will understand the special nature of the management problems involved, which will be quite different from what he is used to in the very unusual circumstances of his psychiatric clinic or office practice. Working with the same psychiatrist over a period of time, the physician may be able to teach him enough about the daily problems of general practice and the life situations of ordinary people who do not consider themselves psychiatric patients for him to be able to get answers which come reasonably close to being useful, but he will usually have to work quite actively to take what the psychiatrist has to offer and to translate it for his own use.

A psychiatrist who has himself had experience in general practice before undergoing psychiatric training sometimes finds this type of consultation easier, but it is surprising how specialized psychiatric training and experience, which dwell constantly on the abnormal and the unusual and on unconscious motivation and irrational fantasy formation, impair the memories of this previous experience with the world of normality. A psychiatrist usually realizes the extent to which this is so and realizes and respects the degree of expertness of the family doctor's specialized knowledge in his own field only after he has been educated by his consultee.

I can vouch personally for the importance of this process because in the course of my own experience in community psychiatry I have been successively educated by social workers, public health nurses, paediatricians, obstetricians, and nutritionists, most of whom were initially a little surprised to find how much they were teaching me during their consultations.

Responsibility for Plan and Implementation

This leads me to my last point. The management plan which emerges from the consultation may have been arrived at as a result of a fruitful joint collaborative endeavour, but the type of plan and the responsibility for its implementation must remain with the family physician and must fit into the general framework of his traditional methods of functioning. Both parties should beware of working out a psychiatrist's plan instead of a family physician's plan and of turning the physician into a 'proxy psychiatrist'. The style of work of the family physician is fundamentally different from that of the psychiatrist.

For instance, take the time relations of their professional work. It may seem that a busy general practitioner would never have the time to make use of the kind of knowledge I have been discussing; he could never spend the time which the psychiatrist can apparently allot to his small select group of patients. This is a red herring. It presupposes that, to cover the same problem, members of the two professional disciplines will use the same approach. This is neither necessary nor desirable, since the different professional roles have been differentiated over a long time in order to cope with problems in a very special way which has been found empirically to be effective and which is recognized by being embodied in the traditional culture of that profession. In this case, for instance, the practices of the psychiatrist in relation to time are based on the fact that his patients are strangers to him; since he has to penetrate below their surface defences and deal with unrecognized and unacceptable material, his relationship with his patient, however intimate the content of their discussions, remains a highly structured stranger relationship, in which each takes care to keep outside the boundaries of each other's customary social life. The regular appointment and the fifty-minute hour are derivatives of this situation, the interview between patient and psychiatrist being specially separated from the rest of the patient's life so as to give him the security to lay down temporarily some of his defences. The length of the usual psychotherapeutic treatment is also dictated by the fact that the psychiatrist has to deal systematically with much complicated material in working down from the surface of consciousness to those hidden areas in which he searches for the unconscious sources of the illness.

The family physician by contrast knows many of his patients as friends. He has known them and their relatives for years, and even in the case of a new patient he can assume that this will be a prolonged contact. He does not need to collect important information about the personality of his patients in a few long highly structured interviews; it comes in dribs and drabs, either directly or indirectly from many and various collateral sources. He penetrates the patient's social life and home as a friend, and very often his patients come into his own home as a friend. Certainly he learns many secret and intimate things about his patients, but the level of such knowledge and the confidence in professional secrecy are such that this rarely leads to a patient feeling the need to hide from the physician in social situations.

Finally, one must realize that, in helping his patient handle emotional problems of the crisis type I have referred to, the family physician does not need to make long speeches. The most powerful interpersonal messages in which one person influences another are often very short. When the time is ripe at the height of the crisis, the right word or the right few words in the right

228

place give better results than a lecture. Often it is a brief aside or an implication of some statement which ostensibly deals with some detail of management of a physical symptom which does the trick. Very often the most powerful messages are conveyed without words – by one's understanding manner, by one's patience, by one's warmth of greeting, or by a sympathetic nod or gesture. These do not take time, and they are the stock in trade of the physician. The results will be determined by their appropriateness in relation to the specific condition of the patient in his current predicament; but if success is only partial the family physician can always rely on being able to wait for additional opportunities in the future, since his relation with his patient will probably be continuing for many years to come. Through his consultations with the psychiatrist, he will gradually become more and more skilful in these areas. I believe that this skill is a main prerequisite for success in preventing emotional illness in our communities.

REFERENCES

BOWLBY, J. (1951). *Maternal Care and Mental Health*. Geneva: W.H.O.; London: H.M.S.O.; New York: Columbia University Press. Abridged version, *Child Care and the Growth of Love*. Harmondsworth: Pelican Books A 271, 1953.

CAPLAN, G. (1954). 'Disturbances of Mother-Child Relationship by Unsuccessful Attempts at Abortion.' *Ment. Hyg.* 38, 670.

CAPLAN, G. (1957). 'Psychological Aspects of Maternity Care.' *Amer. J. Publ. Hlth.* 47, 25.

CAPLAN, G. (1959). *Concepts of Mental Health and Consultation*. Washington, D.C.: Children's Bureau Publication No. 373.

LINDEMANN, E. (1944). 'Symptomatology and Management of Acute Grief.' *Amer. J. Psychiat.* 101, 141.

CHAPTER 9

Comprehensive Community Psychiatry

'Our concepts of patient care are changing. We are
attempting to maintain patients in the local community,
preferably in or near their own homes. We are adapting to
the shortened hospital stay. We are considering how the
discharged patient may comfortably and safely remain discharged. All this indicates the need to intensify collaborative
planning and to improve communication at the local level
so that the patient may have continuity of treatment as well
as the treatment of choice determined by what the patient
requires rather than by what is most easily made available.
There are some examples of this kind of comprehensive programming. But we must continue to work for even more
effective continuous programs that include both preventive
and health protection measures for the well person and good
medical care and treatment for the ill.'

These remarks were made by Dr. Leroy E. Burney (1960, p. 3),
Surgeon General of the Public Health Service of the United
States, when he opened the Conference of State and Territorial
Mental Health Authorities in Washington on 6 January 1960.

At a conference on 'An Approach to the Prevention of Disability from Chronic Psychoses' organized two years previously
by the Milbank Memorial Fund in New York, Dr. Robert C.
Hunt (1959, p. 21) summarized his address on 'Ingredients of a
Rehabilitation Program' as follows:

Q   231

'1. The enormous disability associated with mental illness is to a large extent superimposed, is preventable and treatable.

'2. Disability is superimposed by the rejection mechanisms stemming from cultural attitudes.

'3. Hospitalization as such is an important cause of disability.

'4. The best of treatment-minded state hospitals perform a disabling custodial function.

'5. The custodial culture within a state hospital is largely created by public pressure for security.

'6. Some of the treatment functions and most of the custodial functions of the hospital should be returned to the community.

'7. This can be accomplished only by a change in public attitudes and concepts of responsibility.

'8. Public attitudes cannot be expected to change until hospitals demonstrate the value and safety of community care by becoming open hospitals.'

At the same conference Dr. R. H. Felix (1959, p. 63), the Director of the National Institute of Mental Health, in a paper on 'Legal and Administrative Implications of Rehabilitation', expressed the following point of view:

'I do not mean to imply that we shall soon be able entirely to do away with the problems of social protection which surround mental disorders. Our present patterns are, I believe, too heavily weighted by such considerations, for the majority of patients and in the light of current knowledge, to the detriment of substantive questions of health. Certainly we must find ways to break through the various kinds of isolation, legal, administrative and social, which have traditionally surrounded the treatment of patients with mental disorders. If we can do so, we shall have taken a major step in the reduction of disabilities in this large population.'

232

The opinions expressed by the above authorities draw our attention to the fact that during the past ten years or so there have been converging developments in many parts of the world indicating a radical change in our thinking about community programmes for the treatment and rehabilitation of patients suffering from mental disorders. A few of the workers who have made significant contributions along these lines include T. P. Rees of Warlingham Park, Duncan Macmillan of Nottingham, Joshua Carse of Graylingwell Hospital, and Maxwell Jones of Belmont Hospital, in England; Arie Querido and A. Sunier of Amsterdam, Holland; and Harry Solomons, Jack Ewalt and Walter Barton of Boston, U.S.A.

A consideration of the thinking and the accomplishments of these and other workers leads us to perceive the emergence of a new pattern of community psychiatric care. This pattern is not complete in any one place, but it appears to me that it is already possible, by combining elements which different workers have found satisfactory, to suggest an ideal pattern of a comprehensive programme which may serve as a goal for community planning over the next few years. I propose to describe this pattern and to discuss not only the principles upon which it is based but also some of the methodological and administrative problems with which it is likely to be associated in practice.

PRINCIPLES OF COMPREHENSIVE PSYCHIATRY

The following concepts and assumptions appear to underlie much of the developmental thinking and practical programming to which reference has already been made.

1. *The patient is the focus of the programme.* All treatment, services, and institutions are viewed as interlocking parts of a programme which is designed to meet the current needs of the patient, rather than to try to fit the patients into the institutions in order to satisfy administrative needs or the vested interests of professional groups.

2. *The programme is comprehensive.* It includes primary,

secondary, and tertiary prevention, casefinding, screening, investigation, diagnosis, treatment, and rehabilitation.

3. *The patient is seen as being constantly affected by his interpersonal and social environment.* This is taken into account not only in regard to aetiology but also in regard to casefinding, treatment, and rehabilitation.

4. *Mental disorder is seen as an episode in a patient's life.* The episode may be single or repeated.

5. *The purpose of psychiatric intervention is to return the patient as soon as possible to his ordinary life situation.* It can rarely be the goal of psychiatric intervention to remake the patient into a new person. As a result of his mental disorder the patient departs significantly from his life trajectory, and the goal of intervention is to return him to this life trajectory.

6. *Psychiatric intervention is an artifact in a patient's life.* It should be kept to the minimum in effort and time in order to maximize the possibility of the operation of the spontaneous strengths of the patient and his psychosocial environment. The goal is to obtain the benefit of psychiatric intervention without harming the patient as we have so often done in the past.

7. *Psychiatric programmes should therefore focus on continuous movement of the patient as rapidly as possible through a variety of successive treatment stages to eventual return to the community.* We hope thus to prevent the iatrogenic harms of traditional psychiatric practice caused by separation, isolation, deprivation, incarceration, and the promotion of dependency and regression.

8. *Continuity of therapeutic relationship should be provided from beginning to end of intervention, and if possible in successive interventions.* In order to guide the patient appropriately through the succession of stages of a treatment programme in which he will move from unit to unit, from institution to institution, and from service to service, an attempt should be made to provide him with one or two therapeutic figures with whom he will build

up an enduring relationship and who will maintain therapeutic contact with him throughout the course of this and subsequent interventions.

9. *Treatment should be segmental and not global.* Psychiatric intervention should deal with the current presenting problem embodied in the present episode of mental disorder and as soon as this has been dealt with the patient should be returned to the community. Communication channels between the patient and the psychiatric service should remain open and there should be the readiness to intervene quickly when some other segmental problem of the patient is stimulated by a future life situation.

10. *Active communication must be maintained among all levels of the programme.* Barriers must be lowered between different psychiatric agencies and services, between psychiatric services and community agencies, between the community and psychiatric institutions, and inside the psychiatric institutions. This implies among other things open mental hospitals, full community participation in psychiatric programmes, extensive consultation services, the deployment of significant psychiatric staff-time for community organization and public and professional education and, in general, considerable attention to the co-ordination of programme planning and administration. Since it is natural for any unit to wall itself off, the administration of psychiatric programmes is faced by the important task of counteracting this process and ensuring active communication and its corollary, free movement of patients, of staff, and of messages.

11. *Psychiatric responsibility should extend beyond unit boundaries.* Administrators of all units and services in a comprehensive programme must accept some responsibility for the welfare of a patient not only while he is on their service, but also during his movements before he comes to their unit and after he leaves. The implication is that all psychiatric administrators must interest themselves actively in the affairs of neighbouring agencies and also in community matters.

BASIC UNITS OF A COMPREHENSIVE PROGRAMME

The following units and services form the building blocks out of which a comprehensive community psychiatric programme may be built. The fundamental planning problem will be to ensure the free flow of patients from unit to unit and back again to the community.

1. *The programme starts and finishes with the patient at home within his own family,* although as will be seen later it may be that after treatment for a mental disorder it may not be possible to return him to his own family, and he may have to live in a foster-home or an institution. Both before he enters the psychiatric service and after he leaves, the programme envisages that the patient and his family are the focus of helpful or unhelpful ministrations by a variety of community agencies, with each of which the psychiatric programme must maintain collaborative relationships. These will include educational agencies, recreational agencies, social welfare agencies, public health agencies, religious agencies, rehabilitation agencies such as the Office of Vocational Rehabilitation, medical care facilities including the family doctor and the whole system of clinics and hospitals of the community, etc. In addition to the formal 'caretaking agents' and agencies of the community there is a network of interpersonal relationships of significance involved in those people who have informal roles *vis-à-vis* the patient or potential patient. These include neighbours and friends, storekeepers, bartenders, etc.

2. *Domiciliary Psychiatric Service.* This may be a service operating out of a local mental hospital, out of an out-patient psychiatric clinic, out of a local mental health centre, out of a community mental health centre, or it may be an independent unit. It employs a staff consisting of a psychiatrist, a psychiatric social worker, a psychiatric nurse, and possibly a psychologist, and in ideal circumstances it operates on a twenty-four-hour on-call basis. Members of the team will be ready to go out to a patient's home on an emergency call from the police or from any of the community agencies mentioned above. The primary

purpose of the domiciliary service is to undertake an initial screening in the case of someone suspected of a mental disorder and to make arrangements for initial disposition. Patients may be seen not only at home but in the office of a family doctor or in the emergency ward of a general hospital. Disposition will include referral to an out-patient clinic, to a local mental health in-patient centre, to a community mental health centre, to the psychiatric in-patient service of a general hospital, or to a mental hospital. Disposition might include investigation or treatment of the patient in his home for a short time by the staff of the service.

An ideal domiciliary service not only screens and makes decisions on disposition and referral, but eventually receives patients back into its care after they have made the rounds of the other units of the programme and have been discharged back to their homes. In these circumstances it is responsible for the follow-up supervision of discharged patients by means of visits to the patient's home and by contact with the non-psychiatric care-taking agencies of the community with which the ex-patient may be associated. In connection with its role in follow-up, the service may build up and maintain relationships with industry in its geographical area.

3. *Central Record Room.* The records system is the nerve centre of an effective programme. It should be associated with the domiciliary service. A family record file should be opened at the time of the first contact with the patient. The file should accompany the patient from unit to unit in the programme and should eventually return to the central record room when the patient has been discharged from the treatment system. An essential aspect of a comprehensive programme is that a case file is never 'closed'. At the termination of the current intervention by the psychiatric programme, the file returns to the central record room and is placed in the 'follow-up' category. Arrangements are made for it to be reviewed at regular intervals in order to stimulate the follow-up procedure. It is to be expected that after the termination of the current intervention there will be the need for repeated interventions in the future.

In a large geographical area a comprehensive psychiatric programme may be organized on a decentralized basis. In that case there will be a separate domiciliary service and a separate record room in each district.

In addition to the central file, separate duplicates of portions of the file may be kept in the various units of the programme. Duplicates will also be necessary in the event that a number of patients from the same family are being treated in different units.

4. *The Local Mental Health Centre.* The core of the local mental health centre is a small, in-patient, short-term treatment unit, suitable for the treatment of patients suffering from neurosis and psychosis who can be discharged within a two - to - four - week period. It incorporates facilities for relatively short diagnostic investigations, and it usually incorporates not only an in-patient unit but also an out-patient clinic for the treatment of children and adults, and in many places a day hospital and a night hospital. It may or may not be associated with a domiciliary service and with the preventive services of a community mental health centre.

5. *Psychiatric Out-patient Clinic.* This clinic is designed to investigate and treat children and adults under out-patient conditions. It may be an independent unit or it may be associated with a mental hospital, a general hospital, a local mental health centre, or a community mental health centre.

6. *Community Mental Health Centre.* The main focus of this unit is on extramural services to the community which concentrate upon the primary prevention of mental disorders. The staff of the centre will be deployed within the framework of a variety of non-psychiatric community educational, social, and medical agencies, where they will be available for preventive intervention in relation to crisis situations. For example, the staff may work in a well-baby clinic or a prenatal clinic or on the surgical ward of a general hospital; and they will intervene on the behalf of patients in these situations who are facing life crisis situations in order to help them achieve a mentally healthy adaptation. Such

238

intervention might be focused on individual patients and their families or on groups of people undergoing a common crisis experience as in pregnancy, or as in the case of groups of parents whose children are just entering kindergarten. The other main type of primary preventive activity will focus upon influencing the work of the non-psychiatric caretaking agents of the community – the doctors, nurses, teachers, clergymen, and others. This work will include taking part in pre-professional education and in-service training, and also in providing consultation to these professionals on their problems in handling the mental health dimension of their everyday work.

A community mental health centre is rarely a completely independent unit, but is usually associated with an out-patient clinic for children and adults or with a local mental health centre or a domiciliary service.

7. *General Hospital Psychiatric In-patient Service*. A psychiatric in-patient ward in a general hospital resembles in its functioning a local mental health centre which concentrates on short diagnostic investigations and short treatment of psychotics and neurotics. The advantages of a ward in a general hospital include earlier casefinding through association with the general medical and surgical services of the hospital, possibilities of consultation with other medical colleagues in cases where somatic elements loom large, as in psychosomatic cases, and greater ease of admission in communities where there is still a significant stigma associated with treatment in a separate psychiatric facility. In most general hospitals where there is a psychiatric in-patient service there is also an out-patient clinic which may serve the patients of the hospital and which may also be available for patients who are referred from other community agencies.

8. *The Mental Hospital Admission and Treatment Service*. This service provides possibilities for more intensive and extensive diagnostic investigation than those possible in a local mental health centre or a general hospital psychiatric in-patient service. In these investigations, periods of observation under controlled environmental conditions aid in diagnosis. The hospital also pro-

vides a therapeutic community within the context of which major cases of mental disorder may be treated by a variety of individual and group treatment methods. It is envisaged that the period of such treatment will range from about one to three or four months, but in exceptional circumstances a patient may stay a somewhat longer time in this service.

The admission and treatment service will receive its patients either directly from the domiciliary service or via any one of the preceding units. It will transfer its patients, as soon as their acute treatment has been concluded, to a day hospital or a night hospital, or to one of the other units which will subsequently be described.

9. *Day Hospital and Night Hospital.* These two units may be associated in one building or may be separate. They may be housed on the grounds of the mental hospital admission and treatment service, or in geographical proximity to one of the other units already mentioned. The day hospital provides facilities for a variety of treatment and rehabilitation procedures which are used to treat mentally disordered patients who are able to return home to their families or to a hospital or foster-home at night, because their symptoms do not overtax the tolerance of their environment. The night hospital is designed to provide therapeutic management overnight to patients who, during the day, either may be at work or may live at home or in a hospital or foster-home.

10. *Rehabilitation Service.* This service is primarily part of the mental hospital. It is activated as soon as a patient is admitted and progressively increases its interaction with the patient as he comes towards the end of his acute treatment programme. It includes occupational therapy, recreational therapy, etc., and also in many modern units it includes a 'hospital industries' section in which patients, while in hospital, undertake useful and gainful employment, either in the production of goods and services needed by the hospital, or in contract work for outside industry. The rehabilitation service provides opportunities for vocational testing and vocational training either within its own jurisdiction

or in close collaboration with the Office of Vocational Rehabilitation in the neighbouring community. The service also provides consultation to the domiciliary service, to whose care the patient will be entrusted after discharge, and it is also closely related to the sheltered workshops and supervised industry programme which will subsequently be described.

11. *Services for Patients with Residual Defects.* The new type of dynamic programme should do much to prevent the chronically disabled patient, whom we used to 'manufacture' in our long-stay custodial mental hospitals. Nevertheless, especially in cases where organic pathology complicates the psychiatric picture, it is likely that a small proportion of patients admitted to the programme will manifest some residual blunting of their capacity to adapt to normal community life despite all treatment and rehabilitative efforts on their behalf. For such ex-patients with defects, institutions must be provided which allow them to live in sheltered surroundings and with the necessary nursing assistance, while exploiting to the full their capacities for work and for limited social interaction with the general community. Such institutions will include hostels and 'villages' which will be situated in areas of maximum community tolerance. Experience in many countries, including Belgium, Switzerland, Israel, and England, has shown that there are few patients with residual defects who cannot be provided with an opportunity for some measure of semi-autonomous functioning in the work and social spheres at relatively low cost in such 'open' institutions.

12. *Transitional Institutions.* 'Half-way houses', which are institutions located in the community, have been found to be a useful stepping-stone from the mental hospital, and are of value for some patients who are hesitant in their path to the outside world. Minimal nursing supervision is provided in these institutions and also social support for the discharged patients, as well as casework help, as they explore appropriate paths for their return to social and occupational self-sufficiency.

13. *Foster-Homes.* Some patients who have completed their course of treatment and are well along in their rehabilitation cannot be

returned to their old homes either because of the break-up of their families by death or divorce, or because they may be vulnerable to certain aspects of the family atmosphere, or because they have residual symptoms which would not be tolerated by especially sensitive members of their own families. For such patients, supervised foster-homes may be valuable either as a transition to return to their own family or as a permanent arrangement.

14. *Sheltered Workshops and Supervised Industry.* Sheltered workshops may be valuable either as a transitional device or as a long-term arrangement for patients who emerge from a mental hospital with residual symptomatology or defect. These workshops are usually set up in collaboration with the Office of Vocational Rehabilitation. Some of the best examples of this type of service are to be found in Great Britain, where they have been organized under the jurisdiction of the Ministry of Labour, which has extended facilities, designed originally for the physically handicapped, to ex-patients who have suffered from mental disorders. The term 'supervised industry' refers to industrial firms who in collaboration and in consultation with workers from a mental hospital rehabilitation service make arrangements to employ ex-mental-hospital patients under somewhat sheltered conditions, and with the understanding that they will be free to call for help in the case of any management problem that may arise. In view of the stigma that is still associated with a history of mental disorder in many communities, the way back to self-respecting work often needs to be smoothed in this way.

15. *Psychiatric Social Clubs.* These services had their origin in England nearly twenty years ago, and are nowadays to be found in many countries. They consist of social and recreational centres, membership of which is made up of patients who have completed their treatment for mental disorders, or who are currently in treatment either as in-patients or out-patients. Some professional supervision is provided, but the majority of the club activities are managed by the members themselves. Social alienation is one of the major symptoms of a mental disorder and one of the most

troublesome sequelae, especially in the face of general community attitudes of prejudice against people who have a history of mental disorder. These clubs, in which the shyness and passivity and inhibition of the members are dealt with in a sympathetic and understanding manner by their fellows, form a valuable facility for weaning the alienated ex-patient back to a healthy state of social participation.

16. *Community Organization.* This is listed at the end in order to emphasize that it is not a separate service, but must be an integral part of the functioning of each of the units previously listed. Each unit must actively relate to the community in a variety of ways which may be appropriate to its major goals. Activities will include *public relations* to inform citizens about its work and to stimulate their support for its existence and development; *public education* in order to disseminate information and alter attitudes so that the work of the unit may be facilitated; *organization of volunteers* who will help with the day-to-day management of the unit's activities; and *stimulation of citizen action,* which will include working with voluntary citizen organizations in order to ascertain current feelings of need in the community for extensions of the programme to handle unmet problems, collaboration with citizen's groups to promote legislation in matters pertaining to the prevention, treatment, and control of mental disorders, and collaboration with organized citizens' groups in order to secure the co-ordination of the programme of all agencies in the community that have relevance to the solution of community problems in the health, welfare, education, and religious fields.

ADMINISTRATIVE PROBLEMS

1. One of the basic problems in the administration of a programme along the lines already indicated is that of ensuring the identification of the professional staff with the programme as a whole rather than with an individual unit. Unless this is achieved, it is inevitable that barriers to communication between units will

arise which will result in blocks to the free movement of patients from unit to unit in line with their current needs. One way which has been worked out for dealing with this problem is to arrange for psychiatric and other professional staff to share their working-time among two or more units. Some of the units may need a few full-time staff, but wherever possible units should be staffed on a part-time basis. In order to ensure an adequate appreciation of the problems both of extramural and of in-patient work, an attempt has been made in some places to arrange for psychiatrists to spend about half of their time on each category of activity. This pattern appears to work successfully in the Nottingham community psychiatric programme in England, where the out-patient and other community psychiatric services are staffed by psychiatrists who spend half of their time in the mental hospital.

2. In order to try to ensure continuity of service to the patient during the course of his movements through the system, it is suggested that a junior psychiatrist and a psychiatric social worker should pick up the case in the domiciliary service, and then move with the patient from unit to unit. This can be arranged if these workers distribute their working-time among a number of the units, and also if their working arrangements are kept quite flexible. This pattern too has been successfully tried in Nottingham.

3. Since the personal psychiatrist of the patient is low in the status hierarchy, it is necessary to take special steps in order to safeguard the free movement of patient from unit to unit. Both admission and discharge of the patient at a certain unit will be decided by a psychiatric administrator who because of higher status may overrule the junior psychiatrist, who may be the one primarily interested in moving the patient quickly. In order to overcome this obstacle as well as the many others which will impede free patient flow, it is suggested that a senior psychiatrist in the central administration of the community programme be given the important duty of being responsible for supervision of patient movement. He will be available for consultation by junior

psychiatrists whenever they feel that their patients are being held up, and he will also consult with psychiatric administrators who may feel that the administrative arrangements of their units are being upset by the demands of the overall programme. The supervisor of patient movement will also maintain a checking card-index on all patients in the central record room, and he will systematically spot-check on the duration of patients in the various units so that he can identify those who are being held up in any particular unit longer than the expected period. He will then attempt to remedy whatever administrative or clinical difficulties he may discover at the root of the hold-up.

4. Free entry of patients into the community programme and their free movement throughout the system will depend upon adequate commitment laws. A maximum of voluntary admissions and voluntary treatment should be the major goal; but it is also necessary to pass laws which will facilitate medical determination of eligibility for admission to the programme in those cases where a patient has to be investigated or treated against his will. Adequate safeguards for the patient and for the community can be built into this new legislation while vesting the responsibility for investigation and treatment in the physicians rather than as in the past in officers of the law. In legislative discussions which are currently being held in Hawaii the interesting proposal is being explored of drafting a new law which will admit a patient for investigation and treatment not to a particular institution but to the programme as a whole, under the authority and medical supervision of the Director of the Division of Mental Health.

5. Both investigation and treatment should focus not upon the patient alone but also upon his family. The family must be kept intimately related to the case throughout its course. This is symbolized by opening a family folder rather than an individual case record. It should be taken for granted that in many instances other members of the family will also be involved in investigatory and treatment procedures in their own right and not as contributory factors to the first patient's care. In some cases it is to be expected that siblings or parents may be found to be more

urgently in need of treatment than the person who was originally named as the patient.

6. Although it may be advisable to set up separate in-patient facilities for the investigation and treatment of children, and although specialized staff with training in child psychiatry will be needed in any effective programme, the aim should be to have all-purpose units capable of investigating and treating patients of all ages. The separation of either children or old people for special care in separate facilities places an extra administrative burden on a programme.

7. The smooth operation of this programme will only be possible if the in-flow and out-flow of patients are handled appropriately. This implies building up good working relationships with the other professional agencies of the community which refer patients for investigation or treatment and receive them back after they have left the programme. As mentioned earlier, each unit must be responsible for liaison with relevant community agencies, and if at all possible all members of the psychiatric staff should engage in extramural work, much of which will focus upon consultation with the staff members of the non-psychiatric agencies. The latter agencies should undertake responsibility for handling the mental health dimension of their everyday work and they should increase their understanding and skills by consulting only on occasional cases with the mental health specialists. In addition, psychiatrists should visit relevant agencies on a sessional basis in order to see certain problem cases and help with advice on disposition. Sample cases should be accepted for investigation and treatment by the psychiatric unit in order to explore the practical issues of care for these categories of patient in that particular agency, and in order to maintain liaison and provide material for the education of the consulting psychiatrists. For example, a division of crippled children in a health department, which may be dealing with a thousand new cases a year of children with disabling physical handicaps, all of whom have some form of emotional complication, and many of whom have explicit psychiatric symptomotology, cannot expect to refer a

substantial proportion of these cases to the community psychiatric programme for investigation and treatment. If they were to do so, they would probably take up all the specialists' time, and none would be available for the rest of the community. What is suggested here is that the workers in the crippled children's programme accept the responsibility for handling the mental health component of their regular caseload and that they apply to the staff of the psychiatric programme for in-service training and consultation in regard to occasional cases in order to equip themselves for this task. They might also call in a psychiatrist once or twice a week in order to help them make a more effective appraisal of special problem cases. In addition, they should have the opportunity of referring a few cases each year for full investigation and treatment by the specialist mental health personnel. Thus, they might refer examples of different types of congenital abnormality, a case of traumatic paraplegia, a child who has suffered an amputation after a street accident, and a child with residua of poliomyelitis. Each of these cases, by being made the focus of special study by the mental health specialist, is likely to reveal characteristics of the problems to be encountered in this type of case, which should lead to an improvement in the handling and management of other cases of the same category by the non-psychiatric workers.

8. A major danger for a comprehensive community psychiatric programme is an intake waiting-list. This danger will be reduced if the programme operates on the principle of minimal intervention and maximum use of non-psychiatric community facilities and caretaking agencies in order to distribute the load. It will also be reduced by avoiding stereotyped intake and investigatory practices. An important step in this connection is the abandonment of the traditional 'team approach' to intake and diagnostic investigation. A diagnostic investigation should be no more complicated and time-consuming than the disposition of that particular case at that particular time demands. The traditional team approach in which almost every case is subjected to hours of social history-taking by a psychiatric social worker and a lengthy bat-

tery of intelligence and personality tests by a clinical psychologist, followed by a briefing conference, and then a psychiatric investigation of the patient, followed in turn by another conference which may or may not lead to a decision on diagnosis and disposition, may be a completely unnecessary and unwieldly procedure in order to answer the kinds of question regarding the management of the case which may be relevant. A well-trained psychiatrist, who in private practice will give a diagnostic appraisal and make a judgement on disposition after an interview of one or two hours, suddenly finds himself incapable of similar judgements when he crosses the threshold of some community clinics. He then feels that no legitimate reply on disposition is possible unless ten to fifteen hours of team-staff time have been expended on the case. It is suggested that in an effective programme the psychiatrist should carry out both initial screening and the initial steps of a diagnostic investigation himself. This should include seeing not only the patient but also the family. In many instances he will be able to give an answer to the dispositional problem after half an hour to one hour. In those cases where he deems it necessary, he may decide upon an additional investigation which he will carry out himself or share with his colleagues in psychiatric social work and psychology. The argument that psychiatrists are so over-burdened that they do not have time in community clinics to carry out this initial appraisal cannot be valid, since as a member of the team the psychiatrist traditionally spends at least the same amount of time on the case, except that he does so after his colleagues have put in six to twelve hours' work. The psychiatric social workers' and psychologists' time saved by the new approach can be employed on tasks where their specialized skills can be effective – there is no intention of belittling the use of the 'team', but the demand is made that it be used appropriately.

9. *The problem of 'good cases' and 'bad cases'.* Traditional psychiatric clinics that are individual-patient oriented, i.e. that seek to produce an optimal therapeutic result for those individual patients who by a series of chances are accepted as the focus of

professional work, usually develop criteria by means of which they judge which are the patients for whom their services are most appropriate. Whether or not they are labelled as such, these patients are thought of as 'good patients', since they permit the clinic to achieve its professional goals, either in the area of re-constitution of a patient's personality, or research, or the training of psychiatrists, psychologists, and social workers. If we examine this situation we will realize that in order to be a 'good patient' the individual has to fit the requirements of the clinic. In different clinics such 'good patients' will vary from the child of high intelligence suffering from a reactive behaviour disorder or a neurosis, to the child with a severe schizophrenic psychosis, to the middle-class patient suffering from a borderline psychotic character disorder, etc. Clinics will regard as 'bad patients' those individuals who do not meet their criteria. Thus, some clinics will view as unsuitable patients of low intelligence or who come from low socio-economic-class backgrounds, or patients with alcoholism. Many clinics with staff who are highly trained in analytic psychotherapeutic skills will regard as unsuitable patients with organic brain lesions or those suffering from the after-effects of chronic psychoses.

A clinic that is set up to accomplish high-level professional work and to achieve certain specified goals, whether in the area of treatment, training, or research, is surely entitled to establish such selection criteria for its practice. However, from the point of view of a unit which forms part of a comprehensive community psychiatric programme, this approach may not be very helpful. A large programme might, of course, be able to afford some highly specialized units in which cases of certain types are treated. A decision on this point will depend on the incidence of cases of these types in the community and also upon the supply of professional personnel relative to the prevalence of all cases of mental disorder in that community.

In most cases, however, a clinic that is part of a comprehensive programme must be primarily oriented to the needs of the community and not to the needs of its own workers and its own vested interests as an institution. This means that in such a clini there are no 'good patients' or 'bad patients'. All persons in that community who are in need of mental health help are to be regarded as appropriate clients of the clinic, unless the community programme has designated some alternative unit to deal with them. The onus is then upon the professional staff not to select patients who are appropriate for their customary investigatory or treatment procedures, but on the contrary to try and work out procedures and techniques to accomplish the maximum results in handling the problems of the whole range of cases with which the clinic is confronted and for which the psychiatric programme accepts responsibility on behalf of the community.

10. *The problem of 'swamping'.* Statements such as the above will arouse in the minds of many psychiatric workers trained in the traditional individual-patient-centred approach the fear that a clinic operating along these lines will be 'swamped' by a flow of patients of such magnitude and with such diverse and insoluble problems that high-level professional work will not be possible. The main reason for this fear is the expectation that all patients 'need' lengthy investigation and treatment. If, however, the clinic differentiates not only its methods of intake and diagnosis but also its methods of treatment and management to the specific demands arising out of a patient's current predicament, experience shows that a service for the mentally disordered can keep abreast of its cases just as well as an institution for the physically ill. Many psycho-analytically oriented workers take it for granted that high-quality treatment must inevitably be protracted treatment, because they judge excellence by closeness to the model of psycho-analysis. The best treatment in many cases may, however, be a quite short intervention, and it may not be at all appropriate to belittle this as 'superficial', since it may make as big demands on professional understanding and skill as longer treatments.

As soon as clinic workers realize that they have many alternatives from which to choose, and that once they have accepted a patient they can work out a plan as long or as short as they have the resources to implement, their fear of loss of control of the situation will diminish.

11. *The economy of crisis work.* A community programme organized along the lines suggested here will conserve professional time because patients will be treated during the disequilibrium of crisis periods. During such periods of disequilibrium it has been found that minimal intervention produces maximum lasting benefit. People are more susceptible to influence at such times. If, however, intervention is delayed until the crisis has been spontaneously resolved by the patient and his family, a great deal of professional effort has to be expended in order to get them to re-open the problems and to give up methods of solution which they have already worked out for themselves, but which the mental health specialists feel are not in their best interests.

11. *Research problems.* A new field for research is opened up by this approach. Our traditional psychiatric knowledge in the area of investigatory and treatment techniques is based upon a focus on the long-term, chronic, established case of mental disorder. When we move over to a focus upon a person in the throes of a life crisis, or a patient in the acute stages of the initiation of a mental disorder, or in a period of acute exacerbation of a long-standing condition, and when we widen our focus from one in which the intervention is restricted to the psychiatric specialists and their specialized colleagues to one in which the intervention is to be shared between the psychiatric workers and the non-psychiatric professionals of the community, we realize that there is much room for methodological and technical innovation, and much scope for experimentation and evaluative research on process and results. Research must aim at defining a whole range of investigatory and therapeutic techniques and at working out the details of the characteristics of the patient and environment that should call into play different patterns of professional intervention.

12. *The problem of in-service training.* A major obstacle to the effective implementation of the plan discussed here lies in the fact that the professional personnel to be used have almost all been trained within the framework of a radically different approach. It will take some considerable time before the new approach

filters through to the pre-professional training institutions. It will of course not do so unless the new method has been tried and found to be more effective than the old. The only way to bridge the obvious gap is to institute the new programmes in localities where there is an overall readiness to experiment, and where the professional workers and their leaders are sufficiently flexible to be willing to try to make it work on the basis of judgements that it is necessary to meet the community demands. The success or failure of the programme will then depend upon the degree to which the attitudes and knowledge of the professional staff may be modified by courses of in-service training in order to fit them for their new style of working. In planning such in-service training, maximum use should be made of the services of teachers who have themselves worked in pilot pioneering ventures, and of staff workers who have been sent away for post-graduate training in one of the increasing number of educational centres that focus on the new community approach. Unfortunately, at the present time, and for some time to come, the number of pioneering centres and pilot projects and the number of community-oriented educational programmes will remain small. In many areas it will be necessary for the workers to do their own pioneering development. Some centres have found that it is helpful in these 'bootstrap operations' to set up technical study groups in which colleagues meet together to discuss the implications of their current experience, and in which a mutual learning opportunity is provided rather than the kind of in-service training programme where students gather to receive instruction from a teacher. It has also been found helpful for such auto-didactic discussion groups to meet at intervals in institutes conducted by a consultant from the outside. The latter shares with the group the latest developments from his own pioneering centre or educational establishment, and stimulates and supports continued development in line with local conditions.

13. *Decentralization.* An essential basis for a comprehensive community programme is that there should be close collaboration between the psychiatric service and the non-psychiatric com-

munity agencies as well as intimate links with local citizen effort. This implies organizing the programme in manageable geographical and population units. This is accomplished by decentralization, which is the method worked out to deal with similar problems in the educational, welfare, and general health field. The size of a region will vary according to many local characteristics. In many places units of 50,000 to 100,000 population are regarded as appropriate, but there is much room for experimentation in this connection especially in sparsely settled rural areas and also in large metropolitan areas. Whatever the size and boundaries of the regions, the fundamental local arm of the comprehensive community psychiatric programme should be the domiciliary service, which has the major function of screening and initial disposition as well as eventual follow-up. In a number of programmes local mental health centres are also provided for one or a combination of regions. In future building programmes the distant isolated mental hospitals are of course to be avoided, but since we have inherited many of these from the past, and since it is unlikely that in the United States and Great Britain we will be able to adopt the courageous and revolutionary policy of Denmark and Sweden, which has resulted in the demolition of the huge old buildings and their replacement by smaller modern facilities close to centres of population, we must try to avoid sending patients to the isolated hospitals. We must also do our utmost to reduce the element of isolation by fostering the transport of families to the hospitals and the emergence of the hospital staff into the communities.

CONCLUSION

The programme which comes closest to the ideal discussed above is that of the Nottingham Mental Health Service in England, which serves a population of 390,000 and which includes a mental hospital with 1,078 beds and an extramural system of services which deals with about 2,500 new cases per annum. Dr. Duncan MacMillan (1959, pp. 38–9), the Psychiatric Director of the programme, had the following things to say about it during

253

the discussion of 'An Approach to the Prevention of Disability from Chronic Psychoses – The Open Mental Hospital within the Community' at the Milbank Memorial Fund Meeting in New York, 1957, and I feel that his remarks form a fitting conclusion to this chapter:

'What are the advantages to the patient of such a mental health service integrating the hospital and the community?

'In the first place, under this system of short-term admission the patient can be treated without damage to his self-respect and a proper doctor-patient relationship can be maintained. Continuity of care is provided, and this is done in a flexible way according to the needs of the patient, with the provision of a service to which he can always resort in case of need.

'In the second place, we do not break the interpersonal links between the family and the community which are so important. I became convinced through an investigation many years ago that, no matter how efficient the therapeutic attitude in the hospital, so long as the interpersonal relationships had not been maintained, we had great difficulty in getting the patient home. I feel this is one of the directions in which we must make further progress by treating the family as a unit and not the patient in isolation.

'Third, the hospital becomes a positive factor in the rehabilitation of the patient instead of being, as formerly, an actual barrier to rehabilitation.

'Fourth, the community begins to accept the hospital as a friend in need, and this alleviates the mental torture of the patients upon admission as well as facilitating their return to employment and to the community.

'Fifth, the union of the social community services of the local authority with all the psychiatric facilities of the hospital enables joint preventive measures to be evolved in a way that neither could possibly do separately.

'It might be of interest to mention that I carried out a review of all the first admissions to the Hospital during the year 1954, that is, all those who were first admitted during the year, in order to find out how many were still in the Hospital. I found that only eleven were still in the Hospital. Of these, six are senile cases and one is a child in the children's unit. Not one is a case of schizophrenia. So the community is now locally playing a large part in the rehabilitation of the patient. There were 1,196 admissions in that year altogether, first admissions and readmissions combined.

'The question has sometimes been raised as to whether we are imposing too great a strain on the community. I am quite satisfied that we are not, because our community is a very vocal one and they raise their voice very definitely. Careful evaluation of the degree of strain on the relatives is very necessary in order to maintain a proper balance between, on the one hand, imposing too great a burden on the family and, on the other hand, insuring that the community plays its due part in the rehabilitation of the patient.'

REFERENCES

BURNEY, LEROY E. (1960). 'Opening Remarks' in Conference of the Surgeon General, Public Health Service, with State and Territorial Mental Health Authorities. Washington, D.C.: Public Health Service Publications No. 771, United States Government Printing Office.

FELIX, ROBERT H. (1959). 'Legal and Adminstrative Implications of Rehabilitation'. In *An Approach to the Prevention of Disability from Chronic Psychoses*. New York: Milbank Memorial Fund.

HUNT, ROBERT C. (1959). 'Ingredients of a Rehabilitation Program', ibid.

MACMILLAN, DUNCAN (1959). 'Hospital - Community Relationships', ibid.

Index

abortion, 218
  an attempt at, 29, 174–5
Ackerman, Nathan, 43, 141, 143
'actual depression', 59
administrative action, 3, 7, 11
administrative positions, subordinates and, 144
administrative problems, 243–53
adolescence, 65–6
'affectionless' children, 122
aggression, 62, 126
alcoholism, 249
alienation, 38
alienists, 39
American Journal of Orthopsychiatry (1954), 199
anaclytic, 107–8
anticipatory guidance, *see* guidance, anticipatory
anxiety, 43, 44, 57, 120, 151
  a pregnant girl's, 167–8
  operations and, 52
  pregnancy, 82
  premature babies and, 157
anxiety work, 44–50
apathy, 57–8
apperception, 35
appetite, pregnancy and, 74–5, 215
'Approach to the Prevention of Disability from Chronic Psychoses', 231–2, 254

babies (baby),
  attitude to future, 86–93
  awareness of, 97–8
  fear of malformed, 83–4
  helpless, 113–4
  jumping of, 98–9
  Middlemore's classification of, 58
  premature, 147–57
bereavement, 59, 219–22
Bethesda, 137, 138
blaming, 152
Bleuler, 42
Boston, 5–7, 147, 152
  pregnancy in, 67–8, 75
Boston Children's Hospital, 8–9
Boston Family Health Clinic, 75
Boston Lying-In Hospital, 8–9
Bowlby, John, 3–4, 124, 210, 211
  cit., 120, 121–2, 123
boy, maternal hope for future, 92
breast feeding, 77, 107
Burney, Dr. Leroy E., cit., 231

California, 27
Canada, 137–8
carcinoma, 88
'caretaking agents', 8, 20–1, 196, 197
'carriers', 14, 15, 163, 164, 194
cases, problem of 'good' and 'bad', 248–50

256

Index

support, 140
  during pregnancy, 166–70
surgery, 51–6
'swamping', problem of clinic,
  250
Sweden, 253
symbiotic relationship, 106, 110,
  111, 112, 119
synthesis, 35–6

Tavistock Clinic, 124, 129
teacher role, 179–80
teachers,
  children's problems and, 21,
    197–9
  consultation with, 25–7, 199–
    201
tertiary prevention, viii
thumb-sucking, 177
toilet-training, 100, 102
toxic process, 74
training, problem of in-service,
  251–2
tranquillizers, 223
tuberculosis, 2, 48, 49, 50
Two-year-old Goes to Hospital, A,
  124–8
typhoid, 11–12, 14

ulcerative colitis, 61
umbilical hernia, 125
unconscious, the, 34, 224
urine, pregnancy, schizophrenia,
  and, 70
U.S.A.,
  family in, 9
  pregnancy in, 71–2
  social workers in, 189
  visiting in children's wards,
    211

'villages', 241
visiting,
  in children's wards, 4, 130–1,
    211
  social worker's, in the U.S.A.,
    189
voluntary admissions, 245
vomiting, pregnancy, 87, 88

well-baby clinic care, 109, 111
Whittier Street Public Health
  Center, Boston, 6, 197
work, mother's return to, 128–9
workshops, sheltered, 242
worrying, anticipatory, 50–8
worry work, 43, 44–50